Beyond
Beautiful

Beyond Beautiful

Using the Power of Your Mind
and Aesthetic Breakthroughs
to Look Naturally Young and Radiant

Doris Day, MD

with Jodie Gould

**CENTER
STREET**

NEW YORK NASHVILLE

Copyright © 2018 by Doris Day, MD

Cover design by Jennette Munger. Cover copyright © 2018 by Hachette Book Group, Inc.

Center Street
Hachette Book Group
1290 Avenue of the Americas, New York, NY 10104
centerstreet.com
twitter.com/centerstreet

First Edition: January 2018

Center Street is a division of Hachette Book Group, Inc. The Center Street name and logo are trademarks of Hachette Book Group, Inc.

The publisher is not responsible for websites (or their content) that are not owned by the publisher.

The Hachette Speakers Bureau provides a wide range of authors for speaking events. To find out more, go to www.HachetteSpeakersBureau.com or call (866) 376-6591.

Library of Congress Control Number: 2017951806

ISBNs: 978-1-4555-4258-1 (hardcover); 978-1-4555-4255-0 (ebook)

Printed in the United States of America

LSC-C

10 9 8 7 6 5 4 3 2 1

To the loves of my life and my guiding stars:
Sabrina, Andrew, and Kambiz

———————

"On a day
when the wind is perfect,
the sail just needs to open and the world is full of beauty.
Today is such a
day."

—*Rumi*

Contents

Introduction

Appearance is anything but superficial. Think about the days when you feel your most beautiful. What do you love about those days, and when does that "beautiful" feeling start? Is it with a caress of your soft, smooth skin when you first wake up; receiving a kind word from a friend, partner, or even stranger; or being pleased by your reflection in the mirror? This book is about improving your most important relationship—the one with yourself—in order to be your radiant best and enhance your presence in the world. To achieve these things, you must not think of the mind-body-skin connection as the meeting of three separate entities. Rather, consider that your mind, body, and skin are one and the same. This means that what you see, whether in the mirror in front of you or in your mind's eye, is a reflection of the natural condition of your skin combined with the effects of specific life events and stressors.

When you look tired, sad, or "old," you have a rash, an acne breakout, or flare-up of psoriasis, pay close attention: your skin is also transmitting information about what's going on physically and emotionally. Some stress is heuristic and can work to protect your skin, your body, and your mind, but in many cases it triggers a negative cycle that accelerates aging. It is only through understanding and properly addressing the source of our stress that we achieve lasting results, optimal health, and true beauty. It's not as hard as you might think and I will guide you through, step by step, on your personal journey.

I like to think of myself as a skin whisperer, helping to reveal and enhance skin's beauty by identifying and addressing what's aging it or causing it to look anything less than its healthiest and most radiant. I will teach you how to respond to this information, as well as show you the best ways to treat various skin conditions so you can always be your healthiest, feel your most beautiful, and look your very best.

I've been a board-certified dermatologist for more than twenty years, treating everyone from kids and busy moms (and dads), to celebrities, models, and CEOs. I've also worked in a research lab at New York University and have helped develop several skin care lines for major brands, including Estée Lauder Co. I take health, skin care, and beauty very seriously, and the radical idea fueling my approach is that by being aware of every aspect of our lives—genetics and internal and external stressors—we can change our skin and live the best lives possible. This belief, as well as my studies of philosophy and the humanities, has informed my years of medical practice, journalistic endeavors, and medical research to the acclaim of both my patients and peers.

My techniques are based on the latest scientific understanding of how we age and combine the most cutting-edge, nonsurgical treatments with the best ingredients and supplements to help you age beautifully. You should not consider having another treatment or procedure or buying another product before reading this book.

In addition to being something of a medical detective, unearthing the true nature of my patients' health from the clues their bodies provide, I also consider myself a doctor of self-esteem. Sheryl Sandberg, the CEO of Facebook, advised women to "lean in" in the workplace. Well, I'm challenging you to "dive in" and examine all aspects of your life to understand how they equally contribute to your body and your skin's reflection of you. The results of my treatments have been life-changing for my patients. And now you can experience the same results.

Throughout this book I will show you how to unlock the power of the mind-body-skin connection for yourself, explain the best treatments available, and explore what the future of skin care and beauty holds. I'll share many fascinating stories of patients who have experienced and beautifully overcome many of the same problems you may be experiencing right now. If the advice I gave them helps you, too, I will have done my job.

I know many of you reading this book are searching for the best and most lasting ways to prevent aging, recapture your youth, or freeze time. You are not alone. In a 2017 consumer survey of over 7,300 people done by the American Society for Dermatologic Surgery, nearly seven in ten people surveyed said they were considering a cosmetic procedure. The top three reasons given were: (1) I want to feel more confident; (2) I want to look as young as I feel; and (3) I want to appear more attractive.

Substantial advances have been made that put reversing, and even preventing, much of the aging process well within reach of the average American. We can save the skin from damage, control and complement the repair of existing damage, and improve strength, resilience, tone, and clarity. One method uses the power of nonsurgical approaches to help you look and feel your best, what I call *syringe therapy*. Used correctly, it has great potential to help you age beautifully and look more like the way you feel inside. But used indiscreetly as a weapon against aging, in an attempt to wipe out any hint of a line, wrinkle, or hollow, it can leave you looking older and artificial. Sadly, when I look around, I'm struck by obvious cosmetic mistakes, from overfilled lips and cheeks to clearly missed areas that leave the face looking unbalanced and "done." I call that *syringe therapy gone wrong.*

There are several reasons why a specific treatment may fail. The first is a lack of knowledge. This reason is two-part. On the one hand, science still gives us only a partial understanding of all the processes that age us.

On the other hand is the fact that you can optimize but cannot change your genetics. This means you need to alter your perspective, learning to examine your beauty with the same fine-tooth comb you use to scrutinize your flaws.

The third reason treatments fail is the emotional component. This is problematic when the way we "see" ourselves drives us to change our features, as if changing them alone will change our lives and how we feel about our lives.

And finally, there's ineptitude—unfortunately, there's always someone who's willing to forgo basic aesthetic principles and add a little or a lot, here or there, whether or not you need it, to make a buck. In the hands of these practitioners, the patient ends up looking like a caricature of themselves, and in the worst case, entirely unlike the original version of themselves. I'm here to help you accomplish your aesthetic goals successfully, safely, and effectively.

Do your homework, which you are doing now by reading this book! You should research the experience and training of your physician, get recommendations from friends and other doctors you trust, and, most importantly, don't cut corners. It is very important to see a trained aesthetic physician such as a dermatologist or a plastic surgeon rather than shop for the best price for treatment. It takes years to learn the art of rejuvenation, and continued study to hone the skills. The products themselves do not create the results, just as fabric does not magically fall into place as haute couture fashion on its own. Rather, just as gifted designers craft fabric to fit your body perfectly, we use our tools of fillers and devices to reflate, restore, and enhance your most natural and beautiful self.

A central theme of this book, which I mentioned above, is that there is an emotional component to the way we "see" ourselves, which drives our desire to change our features, as if altering them will also transform our lives.

An excellent example of this came from a woman named Debra who called my radio show, the dermatology show on Doctor Radio, asking about a Botox Cosmetic treatment for her son Jim. She told me and my listeners that Jim was twenty-three, and she casually asked about treatment options to help raise his drooping brows, which she said were negatively affecting his self-esteem. My guest expert, a plastic surgeon, gave a thoughtful account of all the ways the brows could be lifted: through injections of Botox Cosmetic, undergoing a surgical brow lift, and with devices.

I coaxed a little more background information from Debra. I hoped to uncover the internal catalyst driving her son's, and maybe even her own, particular concern. I asked Debra if the appearance of her son's eyebrows had been present since birth, if there was a trauma that had coincided with his brows beginning to droop, and how much her son really minded the look of his brows versus her minding it. She surprised me by replying that the noticeable drooping of her son's brows was present at birth, and the issue was that it made him look like his dad. That caught me off-guard and required further discussion in a direction that was new for me too.

Upon my further, gentle questioning she told me, with great bitterness in her voice, that she had divorced her husband when their son was two. Her husband had since been absent, as well as in and out of incarceration. The picture started to come into focus. It was no wonder this young man was concerned about looking like his father. He may have felt that any resemblance to his dad would make him act like his dad. And given the feelings his mom seemed to have about her ex-husband, as suggested in the tone of her voice, he may also have harbored concern that his appearance could alienate him from her.

My guest and I encouraged Debra to consider how her feelings and her son's fears might be bigger than the physical concern. As we spoke she became increasingly animated, discovering out loud her husband's impact on her son, and how she might have been complicit in allowing her son to feel bad about his features. I could hear the tears in her voice as she recalled the suffering her son had experienced, and as she understood the better path for her son, and even herself, would be to talk about their experience so that, rather than changing his features, they could change what they symbolized. She was so happy they hadn't pursued treatment for the brows before she called in to the show, because a purely physical treatment would not have addressed the underlying issue.

Jim's brow issue illustrates the importance of understanding that looks and personal relationships are deeply reflective of each other. The skin can evoke the glow of love, the burning redness of anger, or the calm serenity of acceptance. As we go along, we'll dig deeper into this connection. I will show you how to identify negative emotions and their potential effects on your appearance, and I'll highlight and help redirect you down the path so you can see and feel the wonderful impact your healthy relationships have on how you look.

"And you? When will you begin that long journey into yourself?"

—Rumi

How you perceive your appearance is not solely about what's external. Before you have a cosmetic treatment, or another treatment or procedure, I want you to consider that there is an internal component driving what you would like to change about your looks. Once you acknowledge it, you'll be able to maximize the benefits of your treatment and enhance your unique, natural beauty with longer-lasting results.

Stressed Out or Stressed for Success?

We all have stress, whether it's at home, at work, or in our social lives. It's an inevitable part of living and not always necessarily negative. Sometimes stress is a natural result of pushing ourselves out of our comfort zone so we can grow and improve in our lives and the lives of those around us. However, recognizing the stressors and how we handle them is what makes all the difference and affects us in ways that we need to understand.

Since ancient times we have used the fight-or-flight response, which produces several hormones, including cortisol, in situations of danger. The fact is, you don't actually have to be threatened to feel that you are. The mind is a powerful tool that can help us handle myriad situations and control our body's response to nearly everything we are exposed to. Over our lifetime, we build millions of memories that are stored in different parts of our brain, immune system, and other organs. These memories affect, for better or for worse, how we respond to situations. What I will help you discern is the direct connection between a particular stressor and the visible physical reaction to it. It's no accident that you are breaking out in sweat, rash, acne, or hives, or shedding hair. Ask yourself: Why is my stress showing up where it is and in the way it is? Why is it showing up now? Understanding the mind-body-skin connection involves getting to the source of your skin problems and finding the best ways to treat it, along with identifying the best treatments available to help the condition clear as quickly as possible.

I'm going to show you how your self-image and specific skin concerns do not form by accident. These issues are deeply rooted. You'll learn how to decipher what your skin ailments really mean— from hair loss and rashes around the eyes, mouth, or hands to acne to how you see yourself aging. I'll also help you employ a mindful approach to healing, to extend the results from any treatments and help you avoid future recurrences of problems. And I'll share practical ways anyone can improve their look, for example, with facial yoga exercises to tone, tighten, and energize your skin. I'll also explain how exercise and nutrition can give your skin that healthy glow.

Your skin is all-revealing, and beautiful, radiant skin equates with healthy skin that is well cared for. You might find that you have an easier time developing and maintaining great skin than others because of genetics, but the better care you take of those genes, the more it will show in your skin.

As we embark upon this journey together, here's my advice on four basic aspects of skin care anyone can follow. Go ahead and give these a try as you read on to discover more about how to be Beyond Beautiful.

Wash: This is the most important step in your beauty and skin care routine. If you don't cleanse, the makeup, pollution, and grime left on your skin can become toxic and aging. I prefer a cleansing brush over using your hands and soap and water. My two favorites are the Olay ProX microdermabrasion kit, which comes with a cleansing brush and is available at any drugstore, and the Clarisonic line of facial cleansing brushes.

Exfoliate: Your skin naturally exfoliates itself but can always use a little help. Exfoliating has been around since ancient times and should be performed regularly on both your face and your body. You can use a chemical exfoliator, like an alpha hydroxy or beta hydroxy acid; or you might choose to physically exfoliate using a scrub or a device. How often you need to exfoliate depends on your skin, the time of year, and the other treatments you're using. Overdoing it will strip your skin and leave it dry and sensitive, so I'll help you understand what's best for your skin as you read through the book.

Hydrate: One of the most important functions of the skin, and essential to life itself, is water balance. When your body is dehydrated, one of the first places it shows is in your skin. This is due to loss of water from the deeper layers of the skin, not just the outer layers. When your skin is dehydrated it loses its firmness, starts to sag, and even looks more wrinkled. In this case you need to hydrate from the inside as well as outside. I have many patients with oily skin that is also dehydrated. They need to improve their water balance but do not need an occlusive moisturizer that will block pores and worsen their acne. Great hydrators include ingredients like hyaluronic, lactic, and phytic acids. These help deliver and hold water in the skin without being occlusive. These acids help to naturally balance the water and oil in the skin, which helps your skin look its best and stay on its best behavior.

Sun protection: This is about prevention. It's always easier to prevent damage than it is to fix it after the fact. No one is excluded from needing sun protection. No matter your skin color or how much time you spend in the sun, everyone needs sun protection and to be sun-smart every day year-round. I'll talk about this a lot more all the way through the book, but you heard it here first.

The ultimate goal is to age gracefully, not helplessly. This is your best chance to take optimal care of your genetic gifts to age naturally and beautifully. I want to help boost your self-image so you can put your best face forward and live up to your genetic potential. Whatever you decide to do next, please don't feel guilty about wanting to take care of yourself. It doesn't mean you're any less serious about or devoted to your other life obligations.

After you read this book, the next time you look in the mirror you'll understand the real reasons for what you see and how to fix what you want to improve. The most important way for you to attain the look you want will be by digging deeper, while also addressing the surface changes to your skin. And remember, you didn't get here overnight, so you don't need to (and probably won't be able to) fix it overnight. Natural and beautiful results take time but are worth it and will last, because they are part of a complete package called YOU!

MY STORY

> "I have found the paradox, that if you love until it hurts, there can be no more hurt, only more love."
>
> —*Mother Teresa*

Everyone has a story—or several stories, good and bad—that affects their lives in powerful ways. Here are two of mine.

At the age of sixteen, my sister Adriane died. She was also my best friend, and in many ways my responsibility, even if I was only eighteen months older. I was the elder sister, but I saw her as prettier, way more self-assured, and wise beyond either of our years. Growing up we shared everything—a room, our clothes, our toys, our records, and our friends. We were inseparable, and while we had the usual sisterly spats, at night we often wound up in the same bed, talking, laughing, and snuggling until we fell asleep.

One day when she was nearly fourteen, she showed me a firm lump in her left bikini fold. She said, "Don't tell anyone." I was frightened by what I saw and could sense that something was clearly wrong, but she made it clear that this was to be our secret so I kept my word and told no one. I was too young and innocent to know how sick she was, and never for a moment thought it could kill her.

Over the next few months she continued to lose weight and experience unexplained fevers, and the lump continued to grow to the point where it was no longer possible to hide from our parents, who immediately took her to the doctors. Within a week the diagnosis of advanced non-Hodgkin's lymphoma was made. She spent most of the next six months in the hospital, where she suffered through agonizing round after round of the most powerful chemotherapy available and high-dose radiation to avoid the spread of cancer to her brain. The result was waves of nausea, intense and unrelenting pain, both from the cancer spreading and from the treatments and tests that go along with it, organ failure, swelling of her body almost beyond recognition—and all to no avail.

One of the moments that stand out to me occurred early in her treatment. I remember going with her to buy a wig for when her hair would fall out from the treatments. Her hair was her pride and joy; it was long and beautiful, and she took great care of it her whole life. She broke down in tears when she saw it coming out in clumps. It caused her as much pain and agony as any treatment she had to endure, and to this day it still brings tears to my eyes to think of how sad it made her. (I treat hair loss in my practice, and I do my best to help anyone else in that same predicament, from any cause of hair loss.) She was wise way beyond her years, and her suffering, through all the treatments, only to die in the end, was a part of her life that I would need years and years to understand and come to terms with.

Losing someone you love takes enormous mental effort and persistence to pry a space between wishing there was a way to erase their suffering and bring them back, and to let the good memories in and to move forward. Over the years, I continued on my own life journey and tried to mask the pain I felt. But it was there and it showed through in its own way, over and over, through a fifty-pound weight gain that was apparent to the world, and in a more subtle but powerful way I saw in my eyes. The most obvious and clear expression of sadness is tears, but I had none. I felt guilty and numb and scared, and I wondered if I was even capable of love if I wasn't capable of shedding a tear over the suffering and loss of my dear sister. Secretly, I also wanted to look older than my years. I know it seems like a strange thing for a young person to wish for, but at the time, I thought that wisdom came with age and it would help me understand what had happened and make it less painful. I wanted to see things differently, and I wanted my lids so heavy they would cover my eyes and my guilt at not being able to save my sister or protect her from harm.

Looking back I know it's because I didn't want anyone else to see how I had failed my sister: failed to keep her safe from harm, failed to support her, to be there for her as she suffered, because I was afraid of what I saw. I now realize these were fears based on the fantasy that I had control over what happened, but I didn't accept this until much later in life.

When I finally hit my rock bottom of despair, fifty pounds heavier and feeling totally alone in the world, I realized I had a choice: I could keep going as I was—lonely, uncomfortably heavy, and sad—or I could do something different. It was time to rise above the hurt and negativity and dedicate my life to something positive, to educating and healing others.

My mission became to honor my sister's memory by doing anything I could to help others see the good in any circumstance, even if there was no good in it at all, starting with themselves.

As an English major at Barnard College, I took courses in literature and philosophy, which helped save my life and shaped my future. My healers were my professors and great writers and thinkers like Kant, Nietzsche, Schopenhauer, Kafka, Mann, Shakespeare, Chaucer, and so many others who portrayed humanity, gave purpose to suffering, and helped me to climb out of my abyss.

I then went on to become a medical journalist, at least partly so I could share my sister's amazing story of strength and dignity and write about hospice care, advocate for quality of life over longevity for its own sake, and explain how illness and medical treatment should involve the entire family, including the individual patient even if they are a child. I also wanted to contribute to changing medical care by becoming a doctor and being my patients' strongest advocate and protector in any way I could.

My love of medicine was also passed on to me at an early age by my father, who was an anesthesiologist. He was a healer and an educator (in addition to being a poet and a wonderful singer). He started practicing medicine during the 1950s and was far ahead of his time regarding his understanding of health, diet, and even skin care. My dad had seen his older sisters age radically at a relatively young age from sun exposure. He was an advocate of using sunscreen and physical sun protection long before it became fashionable. He made sure I never purposely tanned. He also understood the power of nutrition. He always told me, "Never eat after 8 p.m." And science has finally caught up with him. Studies show that if you do all your daily eating within a twelve-hour window, say, between 8 a.m. and 8 p.m., you have a better chance of losing weight and staying healthy than if you consume the same number of calories over twenty-four hours. He also knew the power of exercise and took daily eight- to ten-mile walks.

My dad loved his work and loved sharing his knowledge and seeing the difference that made in others. Sometimes people didn't want to hear that they needed to lose weight or quit smoking, but he found a way to reach them. He taught me to respect the inextricable connectivity among the mind, body, and soul. As a teenager helping out in his office, I remember his saying, "You can't just count on the textbooks—anyone can learn the science. You have to learn how to take care of the person in front of you. Some people are anxious and need you to talk to them about their family and get to know them. They have to trust and have confidence in you so you can take the best care of them with as little medication as possible."

The confidence and calm he instilled in his patients, just by talking and asking questions, is something I incorporate into my own practice. One of the most important lessons my father taught me was how to be a better doctor by treating the whole person. I can help others heal by encouraging them to better understand themselves and learn how to live in the moment.

The credo that I follow is: "For every regret, you should do ten things differently going forward so that regret becomes a blessing." And for all my regrets about not being there for Adriane in the way I wanted to be and wished I could have been, I can open my eyes, now genuinely older and wiser, able to do so many things differently based on what I've learned and experienced, and with gratitude for having had her in my life.

My father taught me the most important lesson in the last weeks of his life. On February 12, 2013, at the age of ninety-one, he was out on one of his daily walks around New York, the city he loved, when he was struck by an SUV that had lost control and swerved up onto the sidewalk and pinned him to the wall near the entrance of Saks Fifth Avenue, on Fifth Avenue and 50th Street, at 11 a.m. on a Tuesday morning. People posted pictures on Facebook of the scene, with comments saying one person was hit and killed. None of us had any idea it was my dad or that the reports were wrong and he was still alive. I got to the ER just as Dad suddenly and rapidly decompensated. He was surrounded by doctors and residents frantically working to resuscitate him. He was dying. I was shocked to see him in such a bad state since just shortly before I had been told he was under observation, alert, and stable. I ran to his side, begged, pleaded with him, and outright sobbed while telling him over and over again, "I love you, I need you, you can't die like this, not now, I still have so much to learn from you!" I was desperate for him to hear me say those words and to hear me thank him for all he had done for me before he died. I knew it meant as much to him as it did to me.

The doctors were kind enough to let me stay. They could see Dad was responding to me; his pressure started to come back up and he came back to life. He survived another seven weeks and was fortunate to have suffered only a minor stroke and no internal injuries. But ultimately his ninety-one-year-old body could not overcome the trauma of all the broken bones, stress, and complications of life in an ICU, even though he was in otherwise excellent health.

In those seven weeks my mom never left his side. My brother and our spouses and children frequently came to visit. I was there every day on rounds helping to oversee his care, ultimately making the choice to accept hospice care to help him pass in peace, knowing how much he was loved and would be missed.

The greatest gift during this time was being able to tell him "thank you" and "I love you" and hearing him tell me he was proud of me and that he loved me. I was so grateful to be able to take care of him and not feel helpless as I had with my sister. I could help direct his care and make sure he was as comfortable as possible. He taught me about dying with dignity and that it is merely a transition, not an end. He told me I saved him, and he said his good-byes to everyone before continuing on his journey beyond this life.

One of my father's proudest moments was when he handed me my diploma at my medical school graduation. He loved that I was a doctor and that I also understood the value of appearance and the impact it had on health. I can still hear so many of my dad's lessons. One of the biggest was him telling me to "first be a woman" when I was becoming a doctor. He would tell me stories that illustrated the importance of balance, and that emphasizing one aspect of life over another was not healthy or fulfilling. He was the ultimate feminist, helping many women become successful in their careers and erasing any thoughts of limits on what they could accomplish. He inspired me in uncountable ways, and his philosophies have impacted who I am, how I treat my patients, and what I believe you can accomplish through this book today.

I didn't choose and had no say in what happened to my sister or my dad, but I chose to define my purpose from the experiences. I want to share in this book some of the wisdom I learned from my father and from my own experiences as a woman and as a doctor. Not only will it serve as a road map to navigating the best skin care and aesthetic treatments throughout the decades, but it will illustrate a whole new beauty paradigm and serve as your homing beacon and GPS as you go through life. In the ten years since my first book, I've honed and expanded my skills as a physician specializing in dermatology and internal medicine. I have traveled the country and the world studying and teaching health and aesthetic vision and treatments. To help advance the science and education of my peers and the public on the art of medicine, I have also served on many advisory boards, on the board of directors of the American Society for Dermatologic Surgery, and taught dermatology at NYU Langone Medical Center for twenty years.

Beyond Beautiful presents a whole new understanding of rejuvenation and the aging process and includes information on the latest advancements in aesthetic ingredients and treatments. It will help you decide what is the best course for you and what to expect and ask your doctor before having any treatment done.

CHAPTER ONE

Look Inside to See Your True Reflection

"And if I asked you to name all the things you love most, how long would it take to name yourself?"

—*Unknown*

Wat makes people beautiful and why? Our subconscious brain sees things that our eyes don't. The furrow of a brow, squint of an eye, pucker of the lips, the way we flip our hair, these are all subliminal expressions of our inner self. They affect the way we communicate and the image we convey to the world. People can make a major change, like reshaping their nose, and not be happy, or they can make the simplest minute change and be thrilled. So much of what we are taught as cosmetic physicians are the individual mechanics of beauty, but the astute aesthetic physician assesses the face as a global aesthetic rather than a set of lines and wrinkles. We understand that faces have complex angles and multidimensional features to be understood and addressed, and we must decipher the subliminal messages that people convey through their appearance, body language, and the words they use to express how they feel about themselves.

My goal is for you to achieve a healthy balance and harmony in all aspects of your well-being. Harnessing the connection between mind, body, and skin will give you control over what you project to the world about yourself through your appearance.

THE NATURAL LOOK

The changes that occur as we age are multilevel and multifactorial. On the deepest level, changes in bone structure, muscle, and tissue make it impossible to appear twenty when you're fifty. This doesn't mean you become less beautiful as you age; it simply means that the balance of your face changes. Beauty at every age has unique value. As you age you need an overall aesthetic blueprint, not a patchwork of treatments, for the best results. I'll give you specific examples of this as we go.

Some patients assume that successful treatment means the complete elimination of all lines and wrinkles, and that if they have a line left, or can still move their forehead, they have more work to do. Patients have been trained to judge outcomes by these extremes rather than encouraged to see the overall improvement. And because we see so many "supersized" cheeks, lips, and bodies, and virtually frozen faces, our vision has become distorted.

As the travesty of Michael Jackson's unfortunate cosmetic surgeries proved, there will always be a physician, or worse, a nonphysician, who is willing to perform a treatment (whether necessary or not) to make money or for other self-aggrandizing purposes. Patients who have too many or the wrong cosmetic procedures end up looking like distorted caricatures of themselves. I want to empower you with the information you need to avoid treatment by an ill-motivated provider.

To enhance your radiance you'll want to seek only an accredited, board-certified expert with the right care. You'll look your best, but everyone will wonder how it's possible that you never change, or they'll tell you that you seem to age backward. And that is a compliment meaning you still look like you!

Take Anne, for example, a once-stunning woman in her fifties, who visited my office not long ago. Her poise, elegant dress, and expertly applied makeup showed that she was sophisticated and cared about her appearance, and our initial conversation revealed that she had a successful career in finance. She hadn't just broken glass ceilings—she had shattered them!

The first thing I noticed about her, however, was that Anne also looked "done." She had no visible nasolabial folds—the lines that go from the corner of your nose to the corner of your mouth. (Guess what? You're supposed to have them!) She had too much filler in her lips and cheeks, which gave her that dreaded "chipmunk cheek" look. Everything about her screamed overdone. I could see she was not working off an aesthetic blueprint but was merely overinflating her face, like a blown-up balloon, to fill every hole and erase every wrinkle. I needed to understand how she saw herself so I could best help her reach beauty goals, rather than continuing on her current patchwork-quilt path of fix-ups.

Was she there, I wondered and hoped, to ask me to correct cosmetic treatments gone wrong? On the contrary, Anne wanted more filler! In her highly self-critical view of herself, all she could see in the mirror were lines, wrinkles, and sagging skin. She was so concerned with recapturing her youth, and everything she thought came with it, that she failed to see the beauty she already possessed.

Of course, Anne is not alone. According to a 2011 poll of 2,000 men and women by *Allure* magazine, a whopping 93 percent of women say the pressure to look young today is greater than ever. One reason is that women tend to compare themselves to the idealized and

Photoshopped versions of models they see in magazines, the movies, and on TV and online.

When we look in the mirror and see two chins instead of one, or worry lines between our brows (we'll address those later), we feel our youth and attractiveness slipping away. What we don't see is how the changes that happen over time can actually add to our beauty rather than diminish it. I want you to get to a place where you can see your own beauty, not just the flaws. If you see only your flaws, don't expect anyone else to see your beauty. This is what I showed Anne and what I will teach you too.

There's no way to rewind time. I am in no way against aging, and I object to the term anti-aging with all my being, but so much of what we dermatologists see is not about time but how it has been spent, such as those days or years of baking in the sun with reflectors and baby oil or the many visits to the tanning salon. Fortunately, there are outstanding treatments to help prevent damage, slow the aging process, and restore youthfulness.

In my consultation with Anne I sought to learn more about her, why she chose to come to me and why at that particular time. She revealed that her husband had left her, without warning, for a woman who was twenty years younger. That had devastated her. She remarked that nearly five years later she was still in mourning, feeling as though she had lost her best friend. She came to see me because her daughter's wedding was coming up, and her ex-husband would be attending with his new wife. Naturally, she wanted to look younger for the encounter.

The more we talked, the more I sensed her sadness and despair. She had gotten married right out of college and had been with her husband for more than two decades. Even worse, she believed her husband would take her back if she only looked younger—as if someone who would trade her in for a younger woman was a catch!

I reminded her of all she had accomplished and that no one could take away her value or diminish her success. When she first walked in my door she couldn't see how remarkable she was; she saw only her flaws and what she felt she lacked, which in her mind was youth. I knew the best way to help her was not only with the aesthetic treatments I could use to rejuvenate her, but also to help her see her true beauty, both inside and out. I convinced her to let me use cosmetic treatments to give her more natural proportions, more reflective of her real beauty. To her great credit, she followed my treatment plan without complaint. I had, as my father had taught me, earned her trust.

While performing these cosmetic procedures, to best help Anne, I also channeled my inner Joel Osteen, the televangelist. I encouraged her to focus on what lay ahead in her life rather than lament what she felt she had lost from her past. I shared with her what I'd heard Joel say about a woman he had met who had also suffered abandonment: "She really didn't need him...She had better things in store for her...I told her, 'That person who left you, they are a weed. Quit watering the weed...Stop feeding your hurt. Feed your future. Feed your destiny. It will make up for the wrongs.'"

Anne had been so busy feeling hurt and loss, she hadn't stopped to think about how special and wonderful she was, how much life she had left to live. But as time went on, she became more involved in activities that interested her and she met someone very special who appreciated her. She later told me she wouldn't take her ex back if he begged. Her life began to come back into focus, and she liked what she saw.

When Anne went to the wedding she felt radiant and confident, and she enjoyed dancing the night away afterward. Best of all, because she was no longer filled with negative and distracting feelings about her appearance, she was able to focus on what mattered most—her daughter.

Sadly, in my work, I often see how the misguided pursuit of unattainable and unrealistic youth and beauty has led people to miss out on enjoying their most endearing attributes and the best days of their lives. Alternatively, a healthy mind-body-skin connection includes gratitude, a healthy lifestyle, being sun-smart, using specific skin care ingredients, and finding the best rejuvenation treatments for you. Once you start loving yourself from the inside out, you'll be able to face the world with a healthier, more beautiful, and more youthful appearance.

WRITE IT DOWN

Here's a tip for monitoring your emotions, which can impact the way you look and feel. Start keeping what I call a "Face Book" journal, where you record your private musings and concerns. Know that less is more in this endeavor. You only need to write a few lines or thoughts. This will help you stick with it over time. You can look back over it every few months to see if you notice a trend or pattern, and in what context, and be better able to understand why you see what you see in yourself and address it in a more lasting way. Before you begin, copy the following affirmations in your Face Book. Read them to yourself every morning when you get up and every night before you sleep; you might even want to carry them with you as a reminder to treat yourself well:

Dr. Day's Daily Affirmations for Loving the Skin You're In

I will look at myself with the kind eyes of a best friend, of someone who truly loves me.

I firmly believe that I have the potential to become my most beautiful self and that my age is something to embrace and celebrate, not erase.

If I have regrets about the past (or present), I will let go of my guilt by doing things differently in the future, turning that regret into blessings.

I am who I am. I accept the things I cannot change about myself.

Keep a Happiness Jar

I learned this from my daughter, Sabrina. Every time something happens that makes her happy—it could be anything, someone smiling at her on the street, something someone says that makes her feel good, a good grade, anything—she writes it down with the date and places it in her Happiness Jar. On her birthday she empties the jar, reads each entry, and starts anew. I hope your happiness jar runneth over every year!

Visiting Your Aesthetic Dermatologist

If you have yet to see an aesthetic dermatologist, here's what the first visit might be like. The first and one of the most important parts of your visit is the assessment.

For me as a doctor, the assessment often starts right when I walk into the examination room. I note the patient's demeanor, as well as their body posture and what I call facial posture, which is their resting facial expression. We discuss any previous treatments and the goals for our work together. I offer a handheld mirror, and together we look at areas of concern and discuss how I would address them. It is important that we have the same vision for the end result; that I understand their goals, and they understand my strategy for helping them reach it.

I investigate every line, wrinkle, asymmetry, and hollow to understand the source so I can create an aesthetic blueprint to address it in the most natural way. Sometimes I need to be indirect in my approach and use more than one product.

For example, lines on the sides of the mouth, extending beyond the marionette lines, are often a sign of teeth grinding. The fix involves using both a neuromodulator to soften the muscles causing the grinding as well as filler to improve the appearance of the lines.

Addressing a specific issue might involve the use of a combination of devices, fillers, and neuromodulators to achieve the optimal results, but less product and fewer visits are needed to maintain the results over time.

BOTTOM LINE

Nonsurgical options for rejuvenation have improved to the point where they can help you age gracefully and look your most beautiful best, in the most natural way, totally avoiding the need for a face-lift. It is important to have a proper assessment, combine treatments as needed, and to always make sure you're in the hands of a trained aesthetic physician, for the best results. And remember, it's not simply about chasing lines and wrinkles; true beauty is about balance and harmony.

The Five Ds

When it comes to facial aging, knowledge is power. Your chronologic age is how long you've been on this earth. The longer the better in this case. Your biologic or physiologic age is dependent on genetics and lifestyle and you have great control over how it goes. It all boils down to the five Ds. I learned about these from my great mentors Drs. Kent Remington and Arthur Swift:

1. **Deterioration:** The loss of collagen, fat, and elasticity, along with surface changes, show as brown spots, redness, enlarged pores, fine lines, deep wrinkles, rough texture, and overall dullness.
2. **Deflation:** This is the loss of collagen and fat, and the remodeling of bone that leads to a sunken or tired look.

3. **Descent:** Deflation and deterioration contribute to descent, although descent can occur on its own. As we age, our hormone levels decrease. This, combined with gravity, genetics, and collagen loss, causes our skin to sag.

4. **Disproportion:** The ligaments that hold everything in place don't change at the same rate the rest of the skin and structures age, which can make your features become out of proportion with time.

5. **Dynamic Discord:** Dynamic discord is the disconnect of your resting expression from your resting emotion, think "resting bitch face." These "Ds" don't sound pretty, but when you add the good "D," *dermatologist*, to the list, you end up with a knowledgeable ally and your best advantage, so that every decade can be your most beautiful. Thank goodness we now have the science and know-how to deal with the five "Ds" of the aging process.

GLOSSARY OF TERMS

Throughout the book I will be mentioning various treatments and terms. Here's an initial list for you to refer back to when you need further explanation:

Neuromodulators

Also commonly referred to as "neurotoxins," a term I try to avoid since it implies making a deal with the devil for beauty. In fact, these are highly understood FDA-approved drugs that are among our safest, most reliable, and most powerful aesthetic tools. They require hours to days to take effect, and about three to four months for the effects to wear off. The most common adverse effects from cosmetic use are bruising and tenderness at the site of injection. In the medication guide for these drugs, there is a long list of possible adverse effects, but they are still among the most thoroughly studied and understood drugs, and with the most scientific publications in medical journals. The reason neuromodulators are helpful is because the muscles of facial expression are powerful moderators of your mind-body-skin connection, helping you emote your true mood, which is very productive and healthy.

Muscles can only pull, they can't push, and for every muscle pulling in one direction there's an opposing muscle pulling in the opposite direction. The laws of physics say you can move in only one direction at a time. When we use neuromodulators to weaken the action of depressors, or muscles that are pulling down, the effect is a lift because the opposing muscles are now in charge and don't have the force of those depressors fighting against them. The best use of these products is to retrain muscles to help create balance and lift, rather than to eliminate expression.

The drugs in this category all have the same active ingredient, but they are biologics, each manufactured differently from a unique source and each with its own special qualities. When this ingredient first became available, we were so excited about what it could do that we took it to the extreme. The result was a lot of frozen faces. Unfortunately, this is still too often done today and the consumer often grades the efficacy of this treatment on whether they completely eliminate motility in the area treated, rather than how they actually look.

As we have advanced our technique and understanding of muscle balance and movement, we have finessed the treatments to help retrain muscles—not freeze them—which is what I like to do for my patients. You want to rebalance, not remove movement, and to create a natural, smooth look rather than a face that looks the same when happy, neutral, or sad.

The drugs are very safe when used properly by trained injectors, but their safety has furthered the false assumption that it's not important who administers them. As with any aesthetic treatment skill, however, training and the aesthetic eye of the provider are everything. You're better off not having a treatment rather than price shopping and having it done badly.

There are currently three neuromodulators FDA-approved for aesthetic use in the US but more, including a topical version, are going through clinical trials and may be available within the next few years. The three currently in use are:

1. **Botox Cosmetic:** The first to be available in the United States, this product is FDA-approved to treat lines between the eyes and the crow's-feet, or lines on the sides of the eyes. Further FDA approval is on the way and should be available shortly for the forehead and possibly other areas. It is also FDA-approved for the treatment of excessive sweating, or hyperhidrosis, and has been a life-changing procedure for many suffering from this condition.

2. **Dysport:** The first to be approved in Europe and the second in the United States, it has a strong following as well. It is FDA-approved for the treatment of lines between the eyes but is used off-label on other areas, as are the other two drugs in this category.

3. **Xeomin:** The third to be FDA-approved in the United States. This is still a niche product, mostly due to little marketing, but it's also an excellent option and is gaining popularity.

Fillers

This is the category of nonsurgical rejuvenation products with the fastest growth and the greatest prevalence of misuse. Fillers are considered by the FDA to be medical devices. They are injected into specific areas of the face, and now often the body as well, with an immediate effect that can last from months to years depending on the product and where it is placed. Too many people take the word *filler* literally and aim to fill lines rather than create lift and balance. Sometimes filling lines is needed and can be very helpful, but it's not the only or, often, the best use of a filler. There are currently thirteen FDA-approved fillers available in the US, and more are on the way. Each has its own special benefits and characteristics, and while there may be more than one in each category, that does not make them equivalent.

Aesthetic physicians study the products, their uses, and placement techniques to make sure we maximize results for our patients, using the least amount of product and in the safest manner.

Hyaluronic acid (HA) is a protein that is natural to your body, and 60 percent of your body's HA is found in the skin. Its job is to hold water, which makes your skin feel resilient and look young. HA can be applied to the skin as a moisturizer, which is great because it will also hold and pull water into your skin. The molecules are typically too big to penetrate skin, though, so if you want a lasting effect, you need to have it injected.

If you were to inject pure hyaluronic acid (HA) into the skin it would last about twenty-four hours—not an acceptable balance for the effort and the cost. Various companies have found ways to stabilize it, so it can last longer, which is essentially what separates one product from another.

I often use a combination of these products on the face for excellent outcomes. Studies show that when done properly, many patients report that they feel they look *more* natural after treatment than they did before treatment. This is because they look more like themselves, more balanced, and more beautiful, but not like they've had a treatment done. It's also because we have a wider variety of fillers and treatments available than ever before so we can address all areas of the face and neck to restore, reflate, and rejuvenate. These fillers can be categorized as hyaluronic acid fillers, non–hyaluronic acid fillers, or permanent fillers.

Hyaluronic Acid Fillers

Lifting Fillers (Juvéderm Voluma, Restylane Lyft, Restylane Defyne): These are usually injected deep, often right on top of bone in the cheeks, chin, along the jawline, and other areas of the face that need more robust fillers to lift and help create contour.

Contouring Fillers (Juvéderm Ultra, Juvéderm Ultra Plus, Restylane, Juvéderm Vollure): These are used in the mid layers of the skin to reflate lost volume and to give balance. They are sometimes layered over the deep fillers or used to soften contours after the deeper fillers are used. Some, like Juvéderm Vollure, are highly versatile and can be used in different layers with different effects.

Airbrushing Fillers (Restylane Silk, Belotero, Restylane Refyne, Juvéderm Vollure): These are great for filling lines and softening the movement that creates the lines. They give a soft, natural rejuvenated appearance without creating that overfilled or "done" look.

Skin Boosters: This is the newest category of hyaluronic acid injectables and is designed to help hydrate the skin (giving it that covered "dewiness"), soften fine lines, and improve skin radiance.

Non–Hyaluronic Acid (HA) Fillers

Radiesse: Made of calcium hydroxylapatite, this product is great for hand rejuvenation as well as for the face and is often used to treat crepiness and lines on the chest. Results can last one year or longer.

Sculptra: Made of poly-L-lactic acid, a material also found in absorbable sutures and designed to help restore your body's natural collagen, this is one of my favorite products for the right candidate. I love what it does for the skin as well as the way it reflates. I use this product for the temples, the entire face, and also for chest, buttock, and arm rejuvenation. It can last two years or longer.

Permanent Fillers

(Bellafill): Polymethyl methacrylate beads (PMMA microspheres) are a nonbiodegradable, biocompatible, man-made polymer. This material is also used in other medical devices, such as bone cement and intraocular lenses. PMMA beads are tiny, round, smooth particles that are not absorbed by the body. When used as a soft tissue filler, PMMA beads are suspended in a gel-like solution that contains bovine (cow) collagen and injected into the face. Skin testing is required before the first treatment to make sure you're not allergic to the collagen component.

Silicone: This is sometimes used off-label for skin rejuvenation and acne scar improvement. Only an experienced, highly trained doctor should administer a silicone treatment. It is not a product I use, or generally recommend, especially now that we have such a broad range of long-lasting fillers available.

Lasers and Devices

I often marvel at the number of lasers and devices available today. I myself have over twenty in my office, and I use them all on a regular basis. Each one has special qualities to help improve skin texture, tone, and health as well as to provide body contouring, fat reduction, and the treatment of stretch marks, acne scars, and other scars. Certain resurfacing lasers also help treat sun damage and lower your risk of developing skin cancer. Lasers and devices are especially useful when used in combination with neuromodulators and fillers. Later I will let you in on my favorite combinations and the best order in which to have the treatments.

Laser: The acronym LASER stands for Light Amplification by Stimulated Emission of Radiation. There are many lasers on the market, some better than others, and it seems that new ones are available on a daily basis. Each uses a specific energy source to create one single wavelength of light, and that wavelength travels in a focused, collimated beam in a single direction. The color or wavelength also has a specific target in or under the skin. Your doctor selects the proper wavelength, energy level, and delivery timing for the target he or she wants to treat. Some lasers target hemoglobin, which is what makes your blood vessels red, and that helps eliminate broken capillaries on the face and body; others target melanin, which is what makes dark spots brown; and others target water, which we use for laser resurfacing to treat overall wrinkling and to improve skin tone and texture and discoloration from excess sun exposure. There are lasers that go deeper and can target fat and others that help stimulate collagen production or tightening of the skin. Using a laser requires special training. Some of the most common issues I see are burns, scarring, and discoloration from inappropriate laser use by inexperienced users.

Pico: Used to break up pigment, erase tattoos, and improve skin tone and texture.

Focused Ultrasound: Ultherapy, as of this writing, is the only device that is FDA-cleared for providing lift to the skin without surgery. It is not a laser but uses high-density focused ultrasound to deliver fractionated heat energy, both superficially and through the deepest layers of the skin to help tighten and lift. It is also approved for treatment of the décolletage, and it is used in off-label treatments for the abdomen, knees, arms, and buttocks as well.

Radio Frequency

There are many devices available that use radio-frequency energy to tighten the skin or melt fat to help contour different areas of the body and treat acne scars, stretch marks, and wrinkles. I explain three of them below.

Thermage: This was one of the first devices of this kind, and there are now other excellent ones available that I will mention throughout the book.

EndyMed Intensif and the Pollogen Legend: These are devices that combine radio frequency with microneedling to help treat lines, wrinkles, stretch marks, and other skin imperfections while also tightening the skin.

BTL Vanquish ME: Multipolar radio frequency is used to help melt fat, tighten skin, and contour without pain.

Coming up...Take the **Mind-Body-Skin Self-Assessment Test** to discover if what you see when you look in the mirror is a true reflection of yourself.

CHAPTER TWO

Through the Looking Glass

(Your Mind-Body-Skin Self-Assessment)

"Sex appeal is fifty percent what you got and fifty percent what people think you got."

—*Sophia Loren*

People often come to me for skin care advice and aesthetic treatments for one of two reasons:

1. To help them look as good and as young as they *do* feel...or

2. To help them look as good and as young as they *want* to feel.

It's important to understand the power and influence that appearance has on your life. This equally includes your perception of your beauty, how you feel, and the reality of your skin's physical appearance. In this chapter we will embark on a journey to tap into the power of your beauty on every level, inside and out.

We all hope to look in the mirror and see smooth, flawless skin and an image of ourselves that compares to an airbrushed cover of a glossy fashion magazine. But when you look in the mirror is the first word that comes to mind "*uughhh*"? If so, you are not alone! You might be surprised to discover that the mirror can sometimes reflect your state of mind more than the reality of your face or body.

By changing the way you view yourself from within, and by leveraging the power of your mind-body-skin connection, you will find many things in that good-looking glass that will make you smile and present your best self to the world. (And, as I will explain later, just the simple act of smiling makes us look and feel better.)

Speaking of mirrors—there is a lot you can do to obscure or eliminate what you don't like about your looks and enhance the true beauty that you possess. I'll help clear the fog so you see only the best and most beautiful parts of yourself; then we'll work to celebrate and enhance those, while minimizing any flaws or weak areas.

There is no expiration date on your face and body. When we examine ourselves in a mirror we tend to zero in on perceived imperfections rather than focusing on our positive traits.

Too often when I hand patients a mirror, their first reaction to their reflection is to cringe or look away. They then point out all their "flaws," and they look at me as if to say, "Is there any hope for me, Doc?" I listen carefully to what they say and look for nonverbal cues to describe how they see themselves. Understanding the full picture of how a patient feels about themselves and why will allow me to treat them in the best possible way.

First and most important, I point out a patient's beauty and the features we should celebrate and enhance. This way, I can help them reach the goal they have in mind, instead of simply taking them from more flawed to less flawed.

I know that no one really wants to look old and wrinkled. We talk about aging gracefully and accepting the process, which is great on paper, but looking old doesn't mean you're aging gracefully, and you can most certainly still be beautiful even if you have lines and wrinkles.

"Here's what I say about aging: It's really scary when you're looking at it from the outside. When you're inside it, it's not scary at all. You feel better."

—Jane Fonda, 78

BECOME A BEAUTY INFLUENCER

Back in the day before people went to gyms, toned bodies were not the trend. The buxom, blonde beauty icon of the fifties was Marilyn Monroe; the skinny-mini Twiggy set the look of the sixties; androgynous-chic was popular in the seventies; the big-haired look reigned in the eighties; and the broad-shouldered nineties were influenced by women in the workplace who thought to achieve career success they needed to look more like men. Check out any TV show or movie from decades ago, and you will see a broad variety of different beauty styles and standards.

Today, however, we have the freedom to be what I call "beauty influencers." We can change the way we look based on how we feel at any given moment in time; there is no one-fits-all mold for what is beautiful. We can have big booties or small ones, yoga arms or arms with jiggle room (as long as that's part of our natural body type and we're healthy on the inside), tats, purple or gray hair worn long or short. Beyoncé, Jennifer Lopez, Mindy Kaling, Sophia Loren, and Meghan Trainor are all considered beauties. None of them is a size 0.

The age bar also seems to be rising, with Jennifer Aniston chosen *People* magazine's "World's Most Beautiful Woman" in 2016 at age forty-seven. The actress, who says she's learned to embrace her appearance over the years, also says that she feels her best when she's healthy and strong. "We've got to really be mindful of what we put inside our bodies and how we sleep and take care of ourselves," Aniston told the magazine.

Sports Illustrated recently made a huge splash with its special swimsuit issue that included the gorgeous plus-size model Ashley Graham (we should start saying real-size instead, because Ashley is the size of most American women). And the breathtaking bikini-clad icon Christie Brinkley appeared in *SI's* 2017 swimsuit issue at sixty-three years young alongside her daughters Alexa, thirty-one, and Sailor, eighteen, proving that age is nothing more than a number. Yes, times are a-changing, along with our attitudes about beauty.

Want more proof that women's way of thinking about their attractiveness is changing? According to a 2016 Allergan survey of 8,000 women from sixteen countries, including Australia, Brazil, Canada, China, France, Germany, Italy, Japan, the United Kingdom, and the United States, the desire to boost self-confidence is now just as important as aesthetics when it comes to beauty treatments. Women are no longer driven solely by the desire to look better, the survey revealed, but by the desire to enhance their appearance and change the way they feel inside as a person. Nearly three-quarters (74 percent) of the respondents said they wanted to look good primarily for themselves (as opposed to wanting to please a husband or partner). It is not surprising (especially not to me, of course) that skin quality is the new beauty ideal and that women around the world are united by an increasing desire to control how they look as time passes.

Take a Self-Compassion Time-Out

Christopher Germer, author of *The Mindful Path to Self-Compassion*, explains that self-compassion can be exactly what is needed to make self-criticism disappear (or at least tamp it down). It is like a safety net that allows you to land gently on the parts of yourself that you're afraid to look at. It might not be an entirely soft landing, but it won't drop you like a trap-door into the depths of despair. It means saying, "I may not be perfect, but

I'm a beautiful person. Perfection is imperfect. I accept my strengths and weaknesses and acknowledge that I have room to improve." It also means seeing yourself as a whole person, not just the parts that the inner critical voice in your head tries to dominate.

Allowing yourself to live in an environment of kindness and warmth, while taking a closer look at yourself inside and out, will make the Mind-Body-Skin Self-Assessment a little easier and less scary.

"Imagine if we obsessed about things we love about ourselves."

—Anonymous

MIND-BODY-SKIN SELF-ASSESSMENT

Think about that quote above, which commonly appears on posters and in many #selfloving tweets. It's nearly impossible to imagine unless you are a narcissist, right? Here's a test that will help you make an honest assessment of your best features, address the areas you'd like to improve (this is the only time when I will say it's okay to examine yourself in a magnifying mirror!), and possibly give you some positive things to obsess about.

First, remove all your makeup and sit in natural daylight. Begin your self-examination at the scalp line and move down to the forehead and then to the brow. (Remember that your left and right will be backward in the mirror.) Divide a sheet of paper into two columns—one for the areas you would like to improve and the other for what you like about your appearance. If it is difficult for you to find something to admire about your face (and body), then you've got to work on stopping the negative self-talk and learn to look at yourself with kinder eyes. Your goal is to make these two columns as even as possible and to eventually have the positive column be longer! Try to catch yourself before betraying your positive self-image—don't sell yourself short!

Here's what Jackie's self-assessment (age fifty-eight) looked like:

COLUMN ONE/NEEDS IMPROVEMENT	COLUMN TWO/POSITIVE FACIAL/BODY TRAITS
My eyebrows are flecked with gray and starting to thin so I have to fill them in on a daily basis. They've fallen so low I have to draw in the arch!	My blue eyes.
	I have long lashes.
My eyelids are starting to feel hooded and slope downward (it gives me a sad look).	My lips are okay—(I secretly wish they were fuller, but I do not like the look of women who have had obvious lip injections).
Forehead lines are getting deeper.	Light complexion (I wish I was olive skinned, but I stay out of the sun and wear SPF 50 sunscreen. I have gotten compliments on my fair skin. It doesn't look too weathered by time).
Earlobes are getting larger.	
My hair is starting to look thin at the crown, and it's getting harder to cover without teasing my hair every day. I hope I'm not going to go bald!	
Hands now show ropy veins and brown spots. I can literally see through my skin—it looks so old and thin!	My legs and butt are still toned thanks to yoga, spinning, and body-sculpting classes.
I have a gummy smile.	I have defined triceps (again, thanks to yoga and weight lifting), but I'm seeing a little floppy skin underneath (not as bad as my grandmother's, which waved like flags whenever she moved).
Freckles (I try to cover with light foundation).	
Deep lines around my mouth.	
My upper arm skin is looking very crepey.	
My most upsetting negative trait—a sagging chin! I call it my "wattle" (I heard about Kybella and am thinking about getting treatment if I'm a candidate).	I have good posture (dance classes as a child taught me to always sit and stand straight). I have to constantly remind myself to straighten up at a computer, however.
I absolutely hate seeing myself in photographs!	

First, congrats to Jackie for coming up with a solid positive trait list! She (and you) will be happy to learn that there is something that can be done to improve each and every negative bullet point! If you are deeply bothered by a physical imperfection that is getting in the way of living your life to the fullest, I suggest ordering your list from most to least troublesome and checking out the chapters here on those issues so you can identify any underlying emotional factors and learn the best treatments available for you. It will not only improve how you look, but, even more importantly, it will change the way you look at yourself and how you present yourself to the world! As you advance through this book, consider your answers to the assessment and you'll find the best explanations and options for each of your concerns.

Above all, choose to see the beauty in yourself. The most beautiful photos I see are when people look relaxed and don't even know the camera is there. It's hard not to pose for a shot, but the more you get caught off-guard, the more natural and beautiful you look. Try to establish an easy, lasting confidence through greater self-acceptance.

"The last of one's freedoms is to choose one's attitude in any given circumstance."

—Viktor Frankl, neurologist, psychiatrist, and Holocaust survivor

---

THE POWER OF BEAUTIFUL THINKING

As I mentioned, the first thing I notice and comment on as my patients and I look in the mirror together is their beauty. To some, their beauty is nonexistent or irrelevant when compared to their perceived flaws.

There is beauty in all of us, and if we don't see it, how can we enhance it? My goal is to first help you see your beauty. I can then show you how to enhance, maintain, and celebrate your best features. This doesn't mean changing how you look; it means looking like the best version of you. And what that version is may change as you age. The ability to tailor your definition of optimal beauty to who you are throughout your lifetime is what I truly consider to be aging gracefully.

Don't Confuse Aging Gracefully with Aging Helplessly

What I've observed during my years of practice is that beauty is a feeling as much as it is physical. It is as much about a life lived to the fullest as it is about the skin that makes up the face.

My greatest fulfillment comes from learning about my patients' lives and helping them see the best in themselves and bringing that to the surface, so that what they see in the mirror is their true beauty. This beauty transcends youth. It is the main reason we can look even more beautiful and radiant at age fifty, sixty, seventy, and beyond.

But living life to the fullest without regard for the well-established science of skin care can have its repercussions. The fact is that up to 90 percent of wrinkles, not to mention uneven skin tone, broken blood vessels, and skin cancer, are results of overexposure to the sun. If you add on even a few years of smoking, decades of stress, and other lifestyle factors, those are the main causes of what you see in the mirror. By making only a few changes, you can turn things around so you like what you see in the mirror.

Great care and attention to detail play an enormous role in enhancing the health and beauty of your skin. Truly aging gracefully means doing what it takes to look your best and believing it's your prerogative to have or forgo aesthetic treatments. When done well, fillers and neuromodulators (like Botox Cosmetic), along with lasers and devices, can truly bring out the best in you, without it looking like you've had anything done. (See chapter 10 for my favorite treatments.)

How you take care of your skin is of great importance. It's never too late to start, and it's never too early, either. Besides sun protection, which I can't emphasize enough (thus, my repeated entreaties), there are other measures that you can take as well. The first step is *proper cleansing*. We all are exposed to pollution, and more and more studies show that pollution is very damaging and aging to the skin. This, in combination with unremoved makeup and the buildup of oils and secretions from skin cells during the day can damage and age your skin while you sleep. If you're out late or too tired to wash your face before bed, or if you're traveling and can't follow your regular routine, you can use a premoistened cleansing cloth instead. But that should be the exception, not the rule. I often use a cleansing cloth to remove makeup and then wash with a gentle cleanser to make sure my face is clean and ready for the next step. It's also a great idea to exfoliate on a regular basis. This can be as little as once every other week if your skin is dry or sensitive, or every three to four days if you have oily, more glandular skin with larger pores.

We've come a long way in creating products to help prevent and treat insults to the skin. My next most important skin recommendation is to *use retinol*. It can be over-the-counter, cosmeceutical or prescription strength, but this ingredient is the most studied and well-understood ingredient in topical skin rejuvenation. It helps build and rebuild the collagen layer, making your skin firmer and younger. It also normalizes skin cell turnover, which helps erase wrinkles and makes your skin more even in tone.

The final step is *moisturizer*. I'll discuss moisturizers in detail later, but as a warm-up, I will advise that you look for ones designed for the part of the face or body you're trying to moisturize. Eye creams are designed and tested for the delicate area around the eyes, night creams add an extra layer to help prevent water loss while you sleep, and many day creams are lighter and also contain SPF to help defend against sun damage.

Completing these simple steps on a daily basis will help maintain optimal skin health and give you the best protection against daily wear on your skin. These beauty tips and the utilization of any of a host of non- or minimally-invasive treatments can help you restore and accentuate your natural beauty.

TEN WAYS TO STOP HATING YOUR FACE AND BODY

1. *If you don't have something nice to say...*

Did your mom ever tell you that? Well, she was right. Whenever you look in the mirror, start by saying something nice. Look for the things that you like about yourself and learn to appreciate your best features. Whenever I get mad at myself and admonish myself, I always add at the end, "But I still love me." Simply saying nice things will make you feel better. I'm starting to see a little hooding on my eyelids and I just tell myself that I like them. Now I have "bedroom eyes"! Don't waste precious energy with negative thoughts that prevent you from making peace with yourself. Old talk, face shaming and body shaming, undermine all of your best intentions and make it impossible to fully enjoy your life and the people you love. Self shaming dulls your creativity and limits the healthy brainpower you need to succeed at work and at home. You've got to fight for your right to love yourself—warts and all (yes, there's a treatment for that).

2. *Never compare yourself to others.*

When you see someone you believe is more beautiful and you think, *I wish I had her legs, eyes, breasts, nose, (or whatever)*, stop yourself. Having the goal to be the same size, the same weight, or have the same features as any other person is unrealistic and sets you up for failure. You have to embrace your unique value.

I know it's hard not to, but don't compare yourself with celebrities or your friends' curated posts on social media. Remember, we are living in a selfie-obsessed, airbrushed, Photoshopped, retouched world.

3. Accept the face and body that your parents gave you and learn to love your "Mom Genes."

According to a 2015 Galderma-commissioned survey of approximately 1,000 American mothers and daughters ages twenty-five to fifty-plus, 77 percent of daughters said they worry about aging like their moms; additionally, more than half of the mothers never discussed aging with their daughters. It's a sticky subject, I know, and, depending on how well your mom has taken care of herself, it can be daunting. This is why Galderma, a skin health company that makes medications and products used in medical and aesthetic treatments, launched a "Mom Genes" campaign to educate women about the genetics of aging and inspire mothers and daughters about the process so they can face the future with more optimism.

You can learn a lot about how the aging process will affect you by observing and talking about what your mom has gone and is going through, including how her skin changed after menopause.

We know far more about aging than our mothers and their mothers did, and you have many more options for treatments and products that can help you maintain your natural beauty. The bottom line: Learn to love your Mom Genes and talk to your mother about your fears (and hopes) for the future, which is also an excellent way to bond.

4. Don't diet!

Take a look at my Beyond Beautiful nutritional plan in chapter 9, in which I explain why foods that are high in antioxidants, such as berries, green leafy vegetables, almonds, walnuts, and fish, can help lower your risk of both skin cancer and premature aging. There are numerous studies that show eating foods high in antioxidants and essential fatty acids (aka healthy fat), will give you added protection against damage from ultraviolet radiation. Nutraceuticals (also known as "functional foods") are specially treated foods, beverages, vitamins, minerals, and herbs that improve your health and your skin. Eating right, regular exercise, and getting enough restorative sleep are your weight control keys to success!

5. Learn to be sun-smart.

This is the single most important thing you can do to prevent skin cancer and premature aging. Use sunscreen with an SPF of 30 or higher every day, year-round, even on cloudy days and even in the winter. A useful trick I use to make sure I cover my entire face is by applying the sunscreen from the periphery, or outside of my face, toward the nose or center. This way I know I'll use more to cover my nose if I need to, but too often I see people feathering the sunscreen out as they get toward the hairline, and that is an area where I see a lot of sunburns and skin cancer. You should also wear a hat, sunglasses, and sun-protective clothing, seek shade, and avoid being out in midday sun when possible. Ninety percent of how your skin ages is within your control and is related to sun exposure and other lifestyle choices. As good as we are with our rejuvenation treatments, it's so much easier to prevent a problem than it is to fix it later. An easy rule to remember is: The shorter the shadow, the more dangerous the rays of the sun. At noon, when the sun is highest, you have no shadow, so your risk of burn and the damage that goes with it is greatest. It's best to avoid outdoor activities at this time if possible, or look for ways to be in the shade. You still need sunscreen all day long, and don't forget to reapply every two hours or more often if you're swimming or sweating it off. Set the timer on your phone to alert you every two hours and always carry sunscreen with you in your purse. It comes in small bottles and powders for the face. Instead of perfecting your tan, learn to perfect your pale!

6.   See your dermatologist for an annual skin cancer screening and evaluation.

Let me make it easy for you. Every year on your birthday, have a check of your birthday suit! Your dermatologist will check for skin damage and cancers and give you guidance about your skin care regimen. She or he can recommend products available at your local drugstore, as well as cosmeceuticals designed to help even out your skin tone, minimize the appearance of lines, wrinkles, and pores, and improve your skin texture. Don't underestimate the power of the right product on your skin. I've seen results that are dramatic and beautiful.

Some of my favorite ingredients are retinol (as I've mentioned), niacinamide, peptides, matrikines, growth factors, caffeine, and vitamin C. One thing you may not know is that the formulation of a product contains two components. The first is the active ingredients and the second is the vehicle. The best active ingredient in the wrong vehicle will either be less effective, completely ineffective, or, even worse, irritating to the skin.

Think of it this way: If you give a pastry chef and a non-baker each eggs, flour, sugar, and butter, who will make the better cake? The chef, of course. As a scientist I look for data and evidence that formulations are effective. I see a wide range of products at various price points that work and others that are essentially useless.

7.   Look first for the latest nonsurgical approaches to rejuvenation.

Remember, the goals are to keep your skin looking its healthiest and to be the most beautiful version of yourself. It's all about baby steps.

It's best to start with great skin care and smaller treatments when you're younger, as needed. The goal at this stage is not to fall behind and have to catch up. It's like making sure there is enough oil in your car so the motor will stay in tip-top shape and extend the life of the car. This is now possible, thanks to the wonderful devices, tools, and products we have available, such as fractionated lasers, devices using ultrasound and radio frequency, soft tissue fillers, and neuromodulators. There's so much you can do, but just as with the formulation of skin care products, these tools are only as good as the training and skill of the person prescribing or administering them. It is very important to see an aesthetic dermatologist so you can get the most out of any treatment you choose.

8. Focus on what you have the power to change.

Rather than spending your energy wishing you were taller or prettier, redirect your focus to something you can change. Tone up by taking a yoga or a Pilates class; learn to play an instrument or to speak another language. Not only will these activities make you feel better, but they will create new neural pathways, which help keep your brain active and younger as well.

9. Surround yourself with beauty.

Creating a beautiful environment at home and in your workspace, or choosing beautiful outfits and accessories for yourself will provide a greater sensual experience, which is what we all crave. Keep fresh flowers on your desk or table, accentuate your sofa with some silk pillows, play your favorite music while cooking dinner, and drink mineral water out of a nice wineglass. It might sound superficial, but studies have shown that environment plays a huge part in our well-being.

10. *Improve your facial posture.*

Throughout my twenty years of practice, it's been very eye opening to watch patents' facial expressions, and what I call facial posture, change as they age. Their brows drop and furrow, lips purse, and cheeks get sucked in. It's as if they are trying to disappear. In chapter 3, I'll show you a great exercise to improve your facial posture.

EVERY WRINKLE TELLS A STORY

In this age of aesthetics, chasing and erasing lines and wrinkles has become increasingly popular, and not just for celebrities. But that doesn't mean it's always a good idea. Not all wrinkles are created equally, and you may be surprised to learn that getting rid of all your wrinkles can actually backfire and make you look older!

Practicing and teaching aesthetic dermatology has been an enlightening journey, partly because it didn't really exist more than twenty years ago. In the past, the notion was "Get old and get a face-lift" or nothing. I've been living and participating in the history of nonsurgical aesthetics, helping to grow the art and the science, which has been very exciting and fulfilling. I confess, my interest is also partly because I'm right there in the prime age-group of women seeking the treatments—so it's really about me too.

One of the biggest and most important lessons I've learned as a doctor is the importance of investigating and understanding wrinkles and other changes in the skin so I can treat the source in a way that will achieve more natural and lasting results. Here's a prime example: One of the biggest wrinkle worries I hear every day concerns forehead lines. For some reason, people hate their forehead lines. It may seem like a simple thing to fix with neuromodulators like Botox Cosmetic or Dysport, but this area is one of the trickiest to treat—and it's never good to completely eliminate the movement that creates the lines.

This is why: One of the most important jobs of the forehead muscle is to lift the brows, which helps keep your eyelids from drooping over your eyes. Chances are, if you start to notice more lines in your forehead, it's because your brows are slowly starting to drop and your lids are getting a little heavy. You probably feel it before anyone else sees it. But the drop often leads you to engage the forehead muscle, to contract it, in order to lift the brow, and because many of the muscles of the face are attached to the skin, the skin moves along with it, which is what creates the forehead lines. The difficult connection for most people to make is that taking away the use of your forehead muscles to lift your brows and open your eyes will actually cause your brows to drop, making them lower and heavier. It will also make your eyelids sag, which is never an ideal situation. In this case, erasing forehead lines might make your skin look smoother, but it won't make you look better or younger. The real solution is to lift the brows, and with the advances in treatments, this can now be done without surgery.

My favorite nonsurgical tightening and lifting treatments are ones that use radio frequency, ultrasound, or laser energy to create heat at specific depths in the skin. These devices stimulate collagen contraction and new collagen formation, which lift the brows or other parts of the face and do away with the need to use the muscle for that action. The result is longer-lasting and more natural-looking. Any remaining lines can be treated with a little neuromodulator and filler to further soften them as needed.

Another example of what I hear on a regular basis is concern over nasolabial fold lines—those lines from the corners of your nose to the corners of your mouth. Women and plenty of men, too, notice those lines deepening as they age and want them treated. Once again, this is easy enough to do, but usually not the best place to start because those lines are often a reaction to deflation of the midface area. By gently and discreetly placing the filler where it's needed, often in the outer part of the cheeks far away from those folds, we can create a soft lift and improve the overall look and balance of the face. This almost always means using a lot less product in the fold itself. The results of this approach are naturally beautiful, and the best part of the magic is that no one will be able to tell anything was done! Above all, learn to love the way you look even more with every passing decade, wrinkles or no wrinkles. I always love a happy ending.

What's Your Skin Cancer Knowledge Quotient?

Are the following statements true or false?

1. A BASE TAN WILL PROTECT YOUR SKIN.

FALSE: Going to a tanning salon to get a base tan for protection against sunburn or sun damage is useless. There is no such thing as a "safe" or "healthy" tan. A tan is a biological, physical signal from the skin that DNA damage has occurred. Enough of that DNA damage leads to skin cancer, premature aging, blotchy and uneven skin tone, redness, lines, wrinkles, and sagging. If you like being tanned, you'd better love being wrinkled! My best advice is to avoid both tans and sunburns.

2. YOU CAN GET SUNBURNED ON A CLOUDY DAY.

TRUE: Even on overcast days, 70 to 80 percent of ultraviolet (UVA and UVB) rays travel through clouds and can cause surprisingly bad burns. In addition, sunlight reflects off snow, ice, sand, and water, intensifying the effects by up to 80 percent. The Skin Cancer Foundation recommends wearing a sunscreen of SPF 15 or higher every day in addition to covering up with clothing, including a broad-brimmed hat and UV-blocking sunglasses—even when it's cloudy.

3. SKIN CANCER OCCURS ONLY IN AREAS EXPOSED TO THE SUN.

FALSE: While skin cancer is much more common in sun-exposed areas, it can occur even where the sun never shines. This is why everyone of every skin type needs a skin cancer screening every year by their dermatologist, from the top of their head to the tips of their toes and every bit of skin in between. I recommend that everyone of all skin types use a sunscreen with an SPF of 30-plus and seek the shade between 10 a.m. and 4 p.m. I recommend an SPF 30 over the SPF 15 to be safe, because I know people typically don't use enough and don't reapply often enough. For more tips, visit www.skincancer.org.

4. THE COLOR OF YOUR CLOTHING CAN PROTECT YOU FROM THE SUN.

TRUE: Not only does the fabric type matter, but, just like with the skin, the color of the fabric affects how much protection it offers against UV rays. Just like sunscreen, the sun protectiveness of clothing can be evaluated and rated with a measuring system called Ultraviolet Protection Factor (UPF). UPF is a similar concept to SPF; however, UPF rates both UVA and UVB protection, whereas SPF rates only UVB protection.

Darker colors, as well as some bright colors, such as orange and red, have higher ultraviolet protection factor (UPF) ratings. Pale and pastel colors have lower ratings. A piece of pale yellow cotton fabric typically has a UPF of 5 to 9, while the same fabric dyed black has a UPF of 32.

When it comes to selecting clothing from your closet, choosing a fabric with a tighter weave that will allow less UV to come in contact with the skin is also very important. You can tell if a fabric is woven tightly by using the "hole effect": hold a particular fabric up to a window or light. The less light you can see, the better the protection.

Many manufacturers offer special UV-absorbing clothes, from swimsuits and shirts to hats and pants. These clothes have special weaves, contain

UV-absorbing chemicals, such as titanium dioxide, and retain their sun-protective qualities after numerous washings and exposure to sunlight.

5. TANNING BEDS ARE SAFER THAN NATURAL SUNLIGHT.

FALSE: The World Health Organization has added ultraviolet radiation-emitting tanning devices—tanning beds—to the list of the most dangerous forms of cancer-causing radiation. The risk of melanoma is increased by 75 percent when use of tanning devices starts before age thirty. New high-pressure sunlamps emit doses of ultraviolet A radiation that can be as much as twelve times that of the sun!

Next...learn why, when it comes to our eyes, we must pay attention to how we see ourselves, which impacts how others see us. Believing is seeing!

CHAPTER THREE

The Eyes Have It—Believing Is Seeing

"When a woman is talking to you, listen to what she says with her eyes."

—*Victor Hugo*

The first thing my patients complain about and want treated (even patients as young as in their early twenties) is the area between and around the eyes. They cringe, furrow, and frown to show me the movement, and they all say the same thing: "I'm very expressive!" I usually reply, with a smile to show my words are at least partially tongue in cheek, "No, that's just being lazy." The reality is, it's impossible for any one expression to convey every emotion you have, but I see people try it all the time! The expressions we make are part emotional and part habitual. There are many instances when people make the same expressions over and over and are not even aware of how or when they are doing it.

My patients are correct in one important way: the eyes are the earliest area of the face to show aging. It's not surprising, considering how delicate the skin is around the eyes and how much wear and tear this very sensitive area of the face is subjected to. As a matter of mechanics, you blink 1,200 times per hour and 20,000 times per day. That alone is enough to cause lines and wrinkles over time. Add in sun exposure, rubbing, and changes in the fat pads, muscles, and ligaments around the eyes, and it's easy to understand why this is an area that shows aging so relatively early in life. This wear and tear also makes the eyes a very complicated area to understand and treat. I see many cases where under-eye filler and eye surgery have changed the shape of the eyes or made the eyes look smaller. There are ways to address this area properly, though, and I will address that in this chapter.

There is more to this area of the face than expression and lines, though. The appearance of the eyes and the upper face relates to genetics, lifestyle choices, how you see yourself, how you think others see you, and even what you hope they don't see.

This happens to be the area I'm most sensitive about in myself, but through learning to understand my own Beyond Beautiful connection, I'm now able to see myself in a more beautiful light.

As a child, the main compliment I remember receiving from the adults around me was that I was "all eyes" and that I had such big, beautiful eyes. But I had my "difficult" years too. One day when I was about twelve years old, I was sitting in the lobby of my building (where I still live to this day) waiting for my friend to come down so we could walk to school together. A young boy about my age from the building walked by, stopped right in front of me, looked me straight in the eyes, and calmly said, "You are so ugly. Do you even see and realize how ugly you are?" It didn't feel good to hear, but he didn't say anything I didn't already feel about myself on some level. I compensated for my feeling ugly by being very athletic, overly nice and friendly, and being as interesting and smart as I could be so people would like me. I often even got the odd compliment that I was much better looking once you got to know me. Thank you—I think. Some of the ways that I compensated for my feelings were productive: I was active, and I studied and worked harder. But some were negative: I was self-deprecating and gave others the impression I was weak and that my friendship could be taken for granted.

It took time and effort to make the needed changes to allow more positive and appropriate thoughts and people into my life. Beauty generates from within and is enhanced by great personal care, gentle treatments, and my relationship with myself and those around me. I see it, and others can't help but notice it too.

The eyes are central to communicating how we are feeling physically and emotionally. When we are sad, sick, tired, or mad, it's usually the eyes that show it first: the same goes for showing joy, love, confidence, and smarts. I can also see the telltale signs of a tough day or a tough year when I look at a patient's eyes. As Harvard-educated author Isaac Lidsky said in his TED talk: "You create your own reality and you believe it. What you see impacts how you feel and how you feel can literally change what you see...What you see is a complex mental construction of your own making."

Your eyes and upper facial expressions betray your feelings. The opposite is also true when you exaggerate your facial expressions in order to emote something you don't fully feel. For example, many studies show that making a facial expression creates the emotion—the same as the expression results from that emotion. The eyes are expressive, and if you want to see the power the eyes have in conveying emotion, watch a cartoon where the characters have little to no facial definition except for brows and eyes, and yet they can convey a full range of emotions through slight changes in the angle of the lids or brows or the way the eyes blink.

I mentioned earlier that losing my sister to cancer when I was a teen affected my eyes. In my mixed-up, grief-stricken young mind, I wanted my lids to grow old and heavy so they would cover my eyes, so no one would see how I had failed her and so I wouldn't see the world without her. Such thoughts consumed me at the time. If you looked at me then, it wasn't wisdom that shone through my eyes; unable to shed tears, it was unspeakable sadness, pain, and a deep feeling of helplessness. It was only when I began to mature and have life experiences, including becoming a mother and a physician, that I was able to literally and figuratively open my eyes to what was really going on inside and stop externalizing my pain. This experience taught me how much we all do this, often subconsciously, and how it can wreak havoc on our appearance and profoundly affect our mind-body-skin connection.

AGING EYES

Deep under the skin is a framework of bone (the skull) and, in the eye area, a socket or hole surrounded by muscles, ligaments, fat pads, lymphatics, nerves, and blood vessels that hold everything together. Each layer and element is important in helping you see, blink, and protect your eyes and vision from harm. The eyes and brows are naturally asymmetrical. The discrepancy becomes more obvious with age as muscle, skin, and bony changes occur. The skin in the eye area ages earlier and faster than the rest of the face, as measured by gene expression—we're talking ten to twenty or more years sooner, which is quite striking.

The components that affect how your eyes age include your DNA, accumulated sun damage, smoking, nutrition, and lifestyle choices, along with repetitive facial expressions. The one thing that doesn't change is what is called the "intercanthal distance," which is the distance from the inner corner of one eye to the inner corner of the other. This is the basis of your overall facial balance and beauty, also called "Phi," which I will discuss in detail on page 89.

COMMON EYE COMPLAINTS

The eye complaints I hear most often from my patients are about dark circles, under-eye hollows, eye bags, crepey skin, wrinkles, drooping of the lids, and thinning of lashes or brows. It's a long list for such a small area of the body, which certainly speaks to the power of the eyes in beauty. Whatever you decide to do, the cosmetic physician must start by carefully investigating the source of each issue before treatment, including any physical or medical causes such as allergies or poor eyesight, which may cause you to squint. Once you discover the root cause of your problem, a combination of skin care, lifestyle changes, devices, and sometimes injectables is often required for optimal, natural, and lasting results.

SOPHIA'S STORY

I saw a patient recently who was a sixty-year-old actress. She had a very strong crease between her brows, even at rest, that would lead me to believe that she was in for a treatment of Botox Cosmetic to help soften those lines. I could see she had beautiful eyes and an especially beautiful smile. Her lips were perfectly balanced, and she had excellent youthful skin quality. When I walked in to greet her, I sat and asked how I could be of help. To my surprise, it wasn't the brow lines she was concerned about. She said she hated the lines around her mouth (what we would call the parentheses). During our conversation her brows were in a permanent furrow and it was hard to avoid noticing, but to her they were invisible. It was clear to me that what she was seeing in herself was not related to anything on the surface. I knew I had to help her see herself and discover the power of her beauty. How did I do this? Through flipnosis, or helping her to see herself the way I did as an aesthetic expert—seeing the best ways to create balance and enhance her overall beauty rather than focusing on her perceived flaws.

We talked about her work and her plans. It turned out she was working hard on a movie script with a team of strong personalities who were all men, all opinionated, and she literally could not get a word out without being talked over. The more we spoke, the more I could see her coming to the realization that her issue was not physical; it was that she literally had to speak up and spew out her words in order to be heard! It was her script and her concept, and she was very proud of it.

As she spoke about the script, her face lit up with a smile, and there was no more furrowing her brows at me. She started to see her beautiful lips and smile, and even agreed that a little Botox Cosmetic for the lines between her eyes would be a great addition. We talked about skin care and sun protection and about the power of facial expression. Mostly, though, we spoke of the power she had over her own work, and brainstormed some ideas for her to take control of the meeting. She let me do the Botox Cosmetic I suggested, with a little filler around the mouth, and she left with a smile: empowered through the mind-body-skin connection and with her beauty enhanced.

DARK CIRCLES 101

Dark circles, those brownish-bluish-purplish clouds under your eyes, are the most obvious signs of sleep deprivation, one too many cocktails, and stress. These dark, zombie-apocalypse shadows can be hard to conceal and are among the most common concerns my younger patients have. What gives the skin under your eyes its color is a combination of blood vessels, pigment in the skin, and thickness of the skin, along with fluid that can accumulate in this delicate, sensitive area.

Here's a list of causes and solutions for dark circles.

1. Not enough sleep.

Solution: Get your beauty rest. Try listening to ocean sounds at bedtime, while taking deep breaths and allowing yourself to let go of your day. Catnaps can help too. We all go through difficult times where we can't sleep, but sleep deprivation is not sustainable over a long period of time.

2. Not enough water.

Solution: You must hydrate. If you're not like me, a person who keeps a water bottle on hand at all times, you can also eat your water because many fruits and vegetables contain up to 90 percent water and, thankfully, that counts toward your needed daily intake. Also use eye creams to directly hydrate the outer layers of this very delicate area of skin.

3. Too much alcohol.

Having one too many can lead to both dark circles and puffiness.

Solution: Try drinking less alcohol and see how magical it is for your eyes. You might also lose a few pounds and feel better as a result of less drinking. All-round, a win-win situation!

4. Allergies.

Dark circles are often a combination of both pigment making the skin darker and redness from dilated blood vessels. Allergies cause increased redness through the latter effect, and rubbing will lead to darkening through increased pigment from the irritation.

Solution: Try to stay ahead of your allergies. If you know what triggers them, take an allergy medicine a week or so before they start or speak with your allergist about how to stay ahead of your allergies if they are difficult to control with over-the-counter treatments.

5. Rubbing.

Every day I see women rubbing and aggressively touching their eyes. It hurts to watch! Rubbing creates a defensive response in the skin, which leads to thickening, wrinkling, and dark circles. It's one of the worst things you can do to the delicate skin in this sensitive area.

Solution: Stop rubbing your eyes! Try gently patting on an eye cream instead.

6. Genetics.

Sometimes our DNA is to blame for dark circles, and while you can't control your genes, you can take great care of your genetics.

Solution: Don't rub your eyes, wear sunscreen and sunglasses, and use excellent products that will keep the eye area as healthy as possible. I'll reveal some of my favorite brands and ingredients later in this chapter.

7. Vascular causes.

Sometimes what looks like dark circles is really the plexus of blood vessels under the skin showing through. Things like rubbing can make it worse.

Solution: Use a firming eye cream or one that reduces inflammation, which can really help. One I recommend is ISDIN K-Ox Eyes. It contains vitamin K and Haloxyl, ingredients that help with puffiness and inflammation, which can contribute to redness. I also like white and green tea extracts in products for the same reasons.

8. Volume loss.

Under-eye hollows create a shadow that can look like dark circles.

Solution: Fillers can be very helpful, but often you need to address the midface before addressing this area directly, and the under-eye is also an area requiring advanced injector technique by a trained aesthetic physician. The product I use most in this area is Restylane. Very little goes a long way and the results are beautiful. But it's not the first area I inject in most patients. Too much filler under the eye displaces the lower eyelid upward and can make the eyes look smaller. Using ingredients such as retinol that help firm the skin is also helpful.

UNDER-EYE BAGGAGE

As I mentioned at the beginning of this chapter, the skin around the eyes is the thinnest skin on our body, which makes this delicate area more prone to the signs of aging than other parts of our face. Additionally, over time, the skin under the eyes loses elasticity and what we begin to see is loose skin called "bags." Couple this with manual stress, such as rubbing and pulling on the eyes or the skin around them, and your bags and hollows can become progressively worse, especially if you have allergies or rosacea of the eyes. Another issue is puffiness. Puffiness can have several causes and one is fat pad herniation, which is usually a genetic problem. A quick test I use in the office is to press on the upper eyelid. If I see a bulge in the lower lid, then I know it's a fat pad issue. If I don't see a change, it's more likely to be fluid, so controlling salt intake and drinking more water should help. To eliminate excess salt from your diet, start by taking the salt shaker off your table. If you're used to adding lots of salt to your food, some dishes may taste bland at first, but your palate will adjust quickly, and you'll soon find that you enjoy the natural flavor of many foods you hardly noticed before.

The second step in curtailing your salt intake is to limit your use of processed and packaged foods. On average we consume 6,000 mg or 1 teaspoon of salt daily, much of which is in the prepared foods we buy at the supermarket. With that in mind, the next time you go shopping, be sure to read the ingredients on the labels, especially on canned soups, crackers, cereals, breads, processed cheeses, canned tuna fish and salmon, cake mixes, and frozen dinners. Manufacturers are required by law to list all their ingredients in order of the most to the least amounts added. You'll be amazed at how quickly your sodium intake will spike to levels far above what you should be getting just by eating processed foods.

Replace salt with flavorful herbs and spices, including garlic, onion, chili peppers, and lemon—the fresher the better. I also suggest going on a fast from fast food, which often contains lots of sodium.

Treatment Options

Surgery: Sometimes the best solution for under-eye bags is surgery to reposition the fat pad.

Devices and lasers: The best noninvasive solutions for eye bags are devices, such as Ultherapy, Thermage, EndyMed, or Fotona Piano Mode, to tighten and lift the brows.

Fillers: Because of the sensitivity of the eye area, most of these treatments, especially fillers, should be administered by a trained aesthetic physician. I often notice volume loss a little lower, in the midface, and start there instead of chasing the hollow of the tear trough or directly under the eye. I find that this approach often makes it less likely to need very much—if any—filler to be placed directly under the eyes and greatly reduces the risk of pushing up against the lower eyelid, which would make the eyes look smaller, make the fat pads look worse, or leave a bluish tint on the skin.

Those who do not want or are not ready for office procedures can try the following home remedies:

Tea Bags for Eye Bags

Want another quick fix for puffy eyes? If you're in a hurry, you can use a tea bag to de-puff in a pinch. Moisten with cool water and apply over the eyes for three to five minutes. It works wonders! Placing chilled tea bags on your eyes will reduce the swelling due to the natural anti-inflammatory properties of the tea. Green tea is the best because it's the least processed and is high in caffeine and antioxidants.

Follow the steps to de-puffing with tea bags below:

You'll need two white, green, or black tea bags, room-temperature water, and a cup.

Put room-temperature water in the cup. Dip two tea bags into the cup for 60 seconds. Take them out and squeeze the tea bags. Lie down and close your eyes. Place the two damp tea bags on your eyes. Let the tea bags sit on your eyes for three to five minutes. This can be repeated twice a day as needed.

Cool as a Cucumber

Here's another great home remedy for under-eye bags.

For this one you'll need black, white, or green tea, honey, and one cucumber thinly sliced into about sixteen slices.

Brew a pot of strong tea (4 cups) and add 3 tablespoons of honey. Let the tea cool to room temperature, add the cucumber slices, and refrigerate 4 hours or overnight. To use: Put one cucumber slice on each closed eye for about 2 minutes. Black, white, and green tea all contain caffeine and antioxidants, the honey is an antiseptic and is soothing to the skin, and the cucumber extract is cooling. Put on calming music and relax. Drink some of the tea you brewed or just plain water. You'll see the difference in your eyes and skin afterward.

Quick-Fix Supermodel Trick

There are many products out now that are effectively a girdle for the skin. They contain polymers that compress the skin under the eye and create a smooth look. The effect can last for two to six hours, and that may be just enough to get you through your day or your event.

CREPEY SKIN AND EYE WRINKLES

Lines around the eyes are often one of the earliest signs women notice of aging, especially "crow's-feet" or "smile lines." Studies show that signs of aging around the eye area can occur for some in their early twenties, with many women showing increased signs of aging around the eyes in the thirties. Makeup is a useful temporary fix. Don't pile on heavy concealer because it can settle into fine lines and actually make the area look worse. Instead, try starting with a great primer and then using a highlighting pen, which reflects light and immediately brightens the under-eye area. If you need more coverage, layer an opaque cream concealer on top, but be sure to warm the product first on the back of your hand so it blends in perfectly.

For more makeup tips, see chapter 10: "Beyond Beautiful Through the Ages."

Treatment Options

Lasers and devices: Fractional lasers work to rejuvenate the skin, and devices that use radio frequency, laser, or ultrasound energy will tighten and lift the skin and target its deeper layers. I now do a non-surgical eye lift with these tools that addresses many common eye area issues to create comprehensive improvement. The result is beautiful, youthful, natural looking eyes that look more open, maintain their shape, and are a true reflection of you!

Neuromodulators: These can be used around and even under the eyes to help smooth the lines. In some cases, especially of those who have had eyelid surgery or who have lazy lower eyelids, neuromodulators can create swelling and can pull down on the lower lid, which is another reason why it's so important to see a trained aesthetic physician. The test we do to see if your lower lid is lazy is called the snap test: we gently pull down on the lower lid, and if it's slow to snap back up, we know not to use a neuromodulator directly under the lower lid.

Fillers: There are exciting new skin boosters and hydrators that can make a noticeable difference in smoothing out the skin around the eyes and the mouth.

Home care: At-home care is as important as any in-office treatment. Eye creams and serums can help minimize the appearance of fine lines and wrinkles, moisturize the skin around the eyes, and reduce inflammation and discoloration. They can even strengthen the delicate skin in this area. Look for eye products with ingredients like caffeine (see the box below), which is an anti-inflammatory. If you have experienced prolonged UV exposure and you are beginning to see fine lines and wrinkles around the eye area, or if you are concerned with aging around the eyes, I recommend using an eye cream sooner rather than later. Some of my favorites:

- *Tensage Stem Cell Eye Cream.* Ideal for the fragile eye area, this cream helps to combat multiple signs of aging around the eyes. Apply before bed to help reduce the appearance of crow's-feet, dark circles, and under-eye puffiness. It contains CellPro Technology, which is a combination of growth factor properties from extracts from the egg of the Crytomphalus aspersa snail, giving potent stem cell benefits. It also includes caffeine, peptides, antioxidants, soothing botanical extracts, brightening agents, and retinol.

- *SkinMedica TNS Eye Repair.* This includes growth factors to improve the appearance of fine lines, wrinkles, skin tone, and texture, and it also contains peptides in addition to vitamins A, C, and E to help support the skin around the eyes, as well as unique ingredients to help improve the appearance of dark circles.

Try makeup products that not only conceal but moisturize. And check the labels of eye creams for ingredients such as vitamins B (niacinamide) and C, and peptides that can moisturize and strengthen the skin around the eye, as well as improve discoloration. I also like retinol for this area, but be sure the products you buy have been specifically tested for the eyes to reduce the risk of irritation. When applying your product, always start at the outer corner of the eye to underneath the eye, then proceed to the inner corner of the eye. This way you are pushing the skin around the eyes upward instead of downward. A gentle patting motion is ideal rather than rubbing.

Wake Up Your Eyes with Caffeine

Many of us cherish that cup of Joe in the morning for its pick-me-up potential—but did you know that caffeine is also good for your skin when included in skin care products?

Here's why:

- Caffeine is known to reduce inflammation, especially in response to UV exposure.
- Caffeine improves the skin's moisture barrier.
- Caffeine increases natural skin hydration components.
- In a study by Procter & Gamble scientists, a caffeine-containing product improved dry skin better than a control product after three weeks of treatment and maintained this advantage over time.

Caffeine is gentle enough to be used on the delicate skin of the eye area, which explains why it is used in many eye products such as the ones below, which I recommend:

- Olay Eye Depuffing Roller
- DDF Advanced Eye Firming Concentrate
- Clinique: All About Eyes Serum
- ISDIN K-Ox Eye Cream
- Restorsea Eye Serum
- Tensage Stem Cell Eye Cream

ASK DR. DAY

Q: *Can you give me your thoughts on EndyMed treatment for crow's-feet? How long does it last and how often do you need it?*

DD: The results have been consistently impressive. The Intensif setting combines microneedling with radio-frequency energy. This can leave redness for from two to five days, but that can easily be covered with makeup after the first day. It has several other settings that use the radio-frequency energy alone to help firm and lift the skin without downtime. It works by heating the deeper levels of the skin to the specific temperature that is optimal for collagen stimulation and tightening of the skin, as well as body contouring. The science behind this treatment is excellent, but the results depend on how much elasticity you have lost. Make sure you find someone who is experienced with it. I use it along with Botox Cosmetic and fillers. Two to four treatments are typically required for optimal results. The neuromodulators are generally repeated at three to five months and the fillers at one year or longer. It's very important not to overfill the under-eye area, because the result can be that the lower lid gets pushed upward, which will change the shape of the eyes and make them appear smaller.

LINES BETWEEN THE EYES

This is the most common area we treat with neuromodulators. There are times I see patients frowning the entire time I'm in the room, without even being aware they're making the expression. The really funny thing is that when I ask them to make the expression so I can see where to treat, they are completely unable to do it; it's a subconscious act and they have to learn how to do it on purpose so they can learn to stop doing it. When I treat this area, and really any area I treat with a neuromodulator, I'm working to retrain muscles, not directly chase the lines themselves. This gives more natural and lasting results and avoids that "frozen" look.

I also teach my patients an important exercise that involves lifting back the ears. This is the opposite of frowning or furrowing the brows, and not only does it help avoid the need for constant office visits, it actually lifts the face and strengthens positive emotions. Here's how it goes:

1. Close your eyes, take a slow deep breath in and out, and as you exhale, feel your face relax.

2. Focus on your ears as you slowly smile; feel your ears lift. Do this a few times, focusing on how the ears move and lift the face as you smile.

3. Now try to lift the ears using those same muscles but without smiling. Once you identify those muscles, do the ear lift, in sets of three, three times a day. I now do this exercise pretty much all day long and have worked hard to strengthen my lifting muscles.

This exercise does three great things: It prevents me from frowning, because the laws of physics say you can move in only one direction at a time, and if I'm moving laterally and outward, I can't be furrowing and moving inward. Second, it lifts the jawline and smooths out my face. And third, it makes me feel happy, the way a smile does; and it makes others perceive me as being open and receptive. Try it! Once you learn how to do it, you'll see that this is the best facial exercise you can do!

DROOPY EYELIDS

Drooping or heaviness of the upper eyelids is often caused by a dropping of the brows or it can be caused by the lids themselves drooping. The underlying cause, which may be genetic, is made worse by lifestyle factors, including chronic sun exposure. This condition can start as early as your thirties, but there are now excellent nonsurgical options that are effective, especially if you start treatment early!

The job of the brows is to lift the lids, but overuse of this expression eventually results in forehead wrinkles, since it's the forehead muscle that pulls up the brow line. Treating the forehead with Botox Cosmetic will easily eliminate the lines there, but the trade-off is that the eyelid problem often worsens because the now-weakened forehead muscles can't raise the brows, and as a result the brows can't lift the lids as effectively. In other words, the Botox makes one problem better, but without treating the source of the condition, it makes another issue worse! Here's what you should do instead for droopy lids.

Treatment Solutions

Tightening and lifting procedures performed on the forehead elevate and situate your brows where they need to be and help your eyelids look and feel less heavy. Treatment with devices and lasers that tighten and lift are ideal and usually result in little to no downtime. I often recommend these in combination with strategically placed neuromodulators to help lift the brows, improve symmetry, and restore the natural arch. Carefully placed, gently removed, eyelash extensions on the corners of your lashes or full fake lashes can also serve to open up the eyes.

THINNING BROWS

The brows frame the eyes and create the balance for the upper face. Unfortunately, like our lashes, our brows can thin as we get older. And also like our lids, they can droop, although for a number of women the brows go up, not down, as they age. For thinning brows I recommend minoxidil, which is FDA-approved to help regrow hair on the scalp and prevent further hair loss. I find it works well for many on the brows as well. As the eyebrows go gray, they can be tinted or dyed. Microblading (similar to tattooing) is also used to add color and give the illusion of increased volume. Eye pencil used with a stencil helps on a temporary basis to shape the brow as well.

Huda Kattan, a beauty influencer, makeup artist, and one of the kindest, most genuine women I've ever met, has an incredible makeup and lash line. With over 21 million followers on Instagram, she is a master at helping women achieve stunning-looking brows and eyes. According to Huda, before filling the brows you should place an eyebrow pencil at the edge of your nose to find where your eyebrow should start. Then use gentle short strokes with your pencil or eyebrow brush to fill in the brows, moving outward toward your temple.

And when it comes to brow-power shape, like me, Huda advises against overplucking. She uses an eyebrow brush to swipe the hairs upward and then trims the ends with small scissors working inward at an angle. You can follow Huda on Snapchat or Instagram @hudabeauty. You also might want to watch our video: https://protect-us.mimecast.com/s/VAqOBAT6zWMu9?domain =yahoo.com.

LASHING OUT

One surefire way to help your eyes look their best is by enhancing eyelashes. The average person has about two hundred lashes per eyelid; they grow in multiple rows and it is normal for the hair to shed every few months as new lashes grow in and push the old ones out. Having long, thick, dark lashes helps hide excess upper eyelid skin and droopy lids, and can make the eyes look more open and enhance your beautiful eye color. Women say that having longer, thicker, darker lashes makes them feel more glamorous and confident.

Here are some of the most common questions I get asked about lashes:

Q: *How will thick lashes enhance my appearance?*
Long, thick lashes make your eyes "pop." Celebrities have been donning fake lashes on the red carpet for years, and now other women have taken notice. Eyelashes have long been a symbol of female attraction (think of batting your lashes as a way to flirt) because they are sexy and seductive. They highlight your eyes, making them look bigger and more gorgeous.

Q: *Why do women's eyelashes tend to thin as they get older?*
Thinning lashes is usually genetic and a natural part of the aging process, but other issues such as hormonal or autoimmune conditions can also contribute to this problem. While thinning eyelashes is normal to aging, just like losing volume in your face (the five "Ds"), wrinkles, and graying hair, there are things you can do to help your lashes grow and look better. Many women have eyelash treatments such as tinting and eyelash extensions, but these can damage the lashes and follicles over time if not done properly.

Q: *What are some basic tips to help women prevent eye problems?*
It's key to remember that we should always start with enhancing and taking good care of what we already have. For example, be extra gentle when removing mascara and eye makeup. If you curl your lashes, do it before, not after, using mascara, and try not to rub or touch your eyes because that can make your eyelashes fall out more quickly. Medical conditions like seasonal allergies can cause itchy eyes and lead to rubbing, which can affect lashes as well as the skin around the eyes.

Q: Can diet, makeup, or improper cleansing cause lashes to thin prematurely?

Taking care of eyelashes and maintaining them should be a daily routine. Fasts, fads, or yo-yo dieting can cause hair shedding and accelerate the aging process, even for your eyelashes. Be careful not to tug at the skin or the roots of the lashes when using eyelash curlers, and always take off your makeup at the end of the day. Use an eye makeup remover before washing your face, and, after washing, pat your skin dry instead of rubbing it.

Q: Is there anything we can do once our lashes start thinning?

Below are some basic everyday things you can do if you notice your lashes falling out:

Brush your eyelashes. There are tiny combs that you can use to brush your lashes before you put on mascara. This helps separate and lengthen the lashes.

False lashes are a fun, quick fix for special occasions but not ideal for daily use because the glue can be irritating to the skin and lashes. And if you rip them off your lids, you can pull lashes out too.

Extensions are another option, but I recommend them only for special occasions since they can put stress on your existing lashes and may cause permanent loss of lashes over time. People tend to overdo it; I've seen some dramatic lash extensions that make me think the person needs to do eyelid weight lifting to hold their eyes open! It's also hard to go back to your normal lashes after having them that thick and long, because it distorts your perception about beautiful-looking eyes.

I often prescribe Latisse to more naturally help grow longer, thicker, darker lashes. This is the only FDA-approved product for this purpose. I was fortunate to be an investigator for the FDA trials for Latisse, so I saw firsthand how well it works. I was impressed with its efficacy and reliability. When you stop using it, your lashes eventually revert to where they were.

Low-maintenance treatments include over-the-counter lash conditioners and primers that can strengthen lashes and are helpful to use under mascara. Companies selling these can't make claims that they grow lashes because that is considered a medical drug claim, but the products can support the growth of lashes, help them look better, and keep them healthy.

Another excellent, low-maintenance option is mascara. It's what most women use to lengthen and thicken lashes. There's an old joke among makeup artists that even women who insist they don't wear any makeup won't leave the house without mascara. There are excellent new mascaras that provide a whopping two to three millimeters of length and also improve thickness. I don't recommend waterproof mascaras for daily use because they are difficult to remove and can even pull lashes off as you do so.

The bottom line on lashes is that they are a simple and powerful way to help you look younger and sexier. If you have time for only one step in your beauty routine, lashes will give you the biggest bang for your effort. Whether it's a temporary or a semi-permanent fix, the eyes have it when it comes to celebrating our feminine beauty.

Browing Out

Try this quick fix for giving your eyebrows more volume from MarieClaire.com. Just rinse your spoolie brush with warm water and rub the bristles on a bar of ordinary soap. Then brush the hairs in an upward direction, being sure to coat each strand with the soap. Finish up with a brow pencil over the coated strands. The waxy texture of the soap builds up and feathers the hair on the brows to give them a fuller look.

Eye Exercises

BLINK

Blinking is a simple way to keep your eyes fresh and helps them to focus longer. When we use a computer or watch TV we tend to blink less, especially when we're staring intently at the screens. Whenever you blink, your eyes produce more tears. Blinking also allows the eyes to go into a brief period of darkness that helps decrease eye strain.

The bright whites of our eyes give us a more youthful appearance. Because redness relief drops tend to be drying, ophthalmologists recommend a lubricant such as Refresh Plus, Retaine, or the aptly named Blink. All are available at your local drugstore, and many eyedrops are available in single-use containers.

THE FIGURE EIGHT

This is a great exercise to strengthen your eye muscles and increase flexibility.

1. Imagine a giant figure of eight (8) about ten feet in front of you.
2. Now turn the figure eight on its side.
3. Slowly trace the figure eight with your eyes.
4. Do it in one direction for a few minutes, and then in the other direction for a few minutes.

BATTLE OF THE BULGING EYES

I see many patients with a special issue of fullness of the eyes, where the eyeballs bulge either slightly or fully out of the socket, which makes them look like deer caught in the headlights. With bulging, the whites above the eye become visible, and that's not attractive. Sometimes bulging eyes are associated with a thyroid condition, and when I see this issue I offer testing to rule out hyperthyroidism.

But most of the time the condition occurs independently of any medical cause. Rather, the eyes bulge outward when a person is literally trying to convey (externally to others and maybe internally to themselves too) their enthusiastic level of engagement by literally reaching out with their eyeballs. The eyes push forward in a show of exaggerated interest and focus. It's always worse when a person is tired, which also shows the world how exhausted or sleep-deprived he or she is and that they're doing everything possible to hold their eyes open.

When I see a patient doing this, I point it out, gently and with kindness, and teach them a facial yoga exercise where they close their eyes and can literally feel their eyeballs relaxing back into the eye sockets. It becomes more effective with practice. I've had patients write letters thanking me for the guidance and advising that they are now able to deal with situations differently because they now understand the mind-body impact on their facial appearance!

WHEN IT'S MORE THAN JUST AESTHETIC

While I'm administering any treatment, I'm also evaluating for possible underlying medical issues. One patient I evaluated was requesting a neuromodulator treatment to help lift her eyes and soften the lines between her eyes. In my assessment I noted that one eye seemed slightly fuller than the other and seemed to bulge just a little, independent of expression. I explained that I often see asymmetry, and it is something I can soften with a neuromodulator. But in her case I also recommended an evaluation by her internist or a neurologist, because I wanted to make sure there wasn't an underlying thyroid or neurologic issue. She thanked me and promised she would follow up as I advised.

When I called a few weeks later to check in, what she said took me by surprise and made me grateful. She said, "You saved my life."

She told me she followed my advice and went to her primary care physician. He scheduled her for a scan of her head, which revealed a brain tumor that was causing pressure on her eyeball. She didn't have headaches, visual changes, or other signs that would have indicated a tumor, but the doctor said it was just a matter of time before the tumor would press on the optic nerve and lead to blindness in that eye. The doctor advised that the type of tumor she had was completely curable and because it had been discovered early, it would be easy to surgically remove. She has since been back to see me on a regular basis for her Botox Cosmetic treatments and has beautiful, perfect symmetry of her eyes.

The eyes play a powerful role in how you view yourself and how others receive and perceive you. My hope is that you have learned from this chapter how to see yourself in the best possible light.

Coming up... *expressive or emotive?*

Are you a lip-purser, a frowner, a smiler, a furrower, or a brow-raiser? Are you most expressive with your face and even your body when you're on the phone? The following chapters will explain how to control your facial expressions, how your emotions can create unwanted lines that seem etched into your face, and how to treat those lines with or without a procedure.

CHAPTER FOUR

Word of Mouth

"The mouth obeys poorly when the heart murmurs."

—*Voltaire*

The single biggest complaint I get from women over forty is about lines above the upper lip. This is one of the most difficult areas to address since we don't want to create an overfilled "duck" look. First, we need to understand what causes these pesky lines. The appearance of aging around the mouth is not caused simply by wrinkles from collagen loss; rather, it is influenced by a complex group of unequal causes, including genetics, sun damage, smoking, lip-pursing, bone resorption, overactive muscles, and teeth shifting. No wonder it's an area of such great concern for so many women! And no wonder it's an area that is often so poorly corrected.

While it is normal for the left and right sides of the face to have some asymmetry, they should be siblings, not twins; the left and right side of the lips, however, should ideally be identical. The lips and mouth area also have important functions like helping to make coherent sounds when you speak, keeping your mouth closed when you swallow or chew, and making facial expressions to help you emote. The mouth area has thirty-six muscles moving in all different and opposing directions, so you can't simply freeze them without ending up looking frozen, drooling when you eat, or not being able to make certain sounds like "p" and "o," among others.

The changes that occur amount to, in the simplest of terms, "deflation," which shows as wrinkles around the mouth; and loss of volume on every level, from bone and shifting of teeth, all the way to loss of collagen in the skin, descent or drooping of the corners of the mouth, and finally, dynamic discord. Dynamic discord is like a resting frown, where the position of your lips sends a message even when they're not moving. The downturned corners of the mouth cause a pouty, grumpy, unhappy look that tells the world something you're not consciously intending to convey.

"Never a lip is curved with pain that can't be kissed into smiles again."
　　　　　　—Bret Harte, American short-story writer and poet

ARE YOUR LIPS SEALED?

Your lips may be sealed, but they not only speak volumes about what's going on inside your head and in your heart, they also have an especially significant impact on how you age in this sensitive area of your face. Here's what the myriad expressions you make with your mouth say about what's really going on with you.

Parted Lips

This can be a look of relaxation, or it can be a signal that you are about to say something.

Pursing/Puckering

Pursed lips are one of the most common over-expressions I see in my practice in women who complain of lip lines. The orbicularis oris is a round muscle that surrounds your lips and mouth, and when engaged, it closes like a purse string, forcing your lips together and creating those annoying lip lines over time. Following are some possibilities of what could be making the lines around your mouth more pronounced for your age. Think about whether or not any of these statements ring true for you and if they are contributing to your expression lines:

- You're hiding teeth you wish were lighter in color or prettier.

- You are suppressing your annoyance.

- You are having trouble making a decision. Further signs of uncertainty are when someone touches their lips with their fingers.

There is much that can be done to treat these lines, though a combination of devices like Ultherapy and EndyMed Intensif, or microneedling, along with a neuromodulator and the airbrushing types of fillers like Volbella, Belotero, and Restylane Silk is often required. The results are beautiful, long-lasting, and very natural-looking, though, when treatment is administered by a trained aesthetic physician.

Flattening Lips

Lips tend to flatten and deflate with age, and the newer fillers, such as Restylane Silk and Volbella, are excellent products for reshaping without overfilling. Lips that are kept horizontal but squeezed flat in an exaggerated closing of the mouth, sometimes called the "lip press," may be simply a matter of anatomy, a sign of uneven dentition and poor support of the teeth and the lips. If we dig a little deeper, however, on an emotional level this action may also be a sign of repressing a desire to speak. Some of my patients worry that "if I spoke, I would be perceived as overly critical." Flattened lips may also be an expression of depression and holding back an impulse to cry. Turning down the corners of the mouth can be a nonverbal expression of sadness. All of these clues are hints not absolutes, and understanding them helps give lasting and meaningful results.

Biting and Lip Licking

Biting the lip in the center or at the side, usually of the bottom lip, is a clear sign of anxiety. Lip biting can become a bad habit or a tic, and people will often do this in certain predictable situations, such as when public speaking or when put on the spot about something. Lip licking might simply be a bad habit from trying to moisten dry lips, or a fairly childlike reaction to stress. Lip biting and lip licking also serve as comforting actions for some when nervous, or as yet another way of suppressing oneself from expressing thoughts and feelings.

Gummy Smile

When you smile do your gums show? If so, you'll be pleased to know that this can be treated with a neuromodulator alone or in combination with fillers and paying attention to the way you smile.

There are two types of gummy smiles: one where the entire top lip rises and shortens the distance from the upper lip to the nose, which exposes gums; and the other where the upper lip actually rolls under when one smiles. If you take a photo of yourself at rest and then smiling, you will be able to see the difference.

The injections needed to correct each type of gummy smile are very different. This is not a well-known procedure for many aesthetic physicians. You may need to be your own advocate when talking to your doctor or finding one who knows how to treat these different types of gummy smiles.

Relaxed

Finally, the lips will be in a position of rest when they are not pulled in any direction. We usually do this when we are feeling most at ease.

PREVENTION

One of the keys to improving your appearance naturally is learning how to recognize the ways your facial expressions affect how you look and feel. The face conveys a universal system of signals that reflect as well as influence your emotional state. Practicing control of your facial expressions will help to improve your appearance as well as how you feel.

To prevent wrinkles around the mouth, take a moment to completely relax your face and then let yourself laugh and be authentic with your feelings. Try taking the Smile Test below.

The Smile Test

Did you know that most smiles are asymmetrical? Most people's facial muscles are stronger on one side of the face than the other. One brow goes up more and one side of the mouth rises higher than the other in a smile. This can also make the cheeks look unbalanced and the nasolabial fold on the stronger side look deeper. Take out the mirror again and think about something funny that will make you genuinely smile to see which side is stronger in you. Now focus on the weaker side and practice smiling harder from that side. When you look in the mirror, you can see the balance, so even if it feels strange at first you will know it looks normal and you'll be able to re-create a more balanced smile.

SOMETHING TO SMILE ABOUT

Your teeth support your lips and help them look more symmetrical and fuller. As you age, your teeth can shift and bone loss can occur, which will make the lips look deflated and uneven, and may even contribute to upper lip lines. This is because as your chin recedes, especially if you have an overbite, more movement and energy are required to put your lips together and close your mouth. That pursing action exacerbates the lines around the mouth. If you grind your teeth, which many people do in their sleep, the muscles that help you chew often overgrow and also cause shifting of your teeth.

There are several options for improving teeth. My husband, Michael Ghalili, DDS, DMD, is a brilliant cosmetic dentist, and he has taught me that there are excellent options available, such as Invisalign and veneers, for improving the appearance of misaligned teeth. There are also "no-prep veneers," so you don't have to file down the teeth beforehand; rather, you simply place the veneers on top of the tooth surface, and they look as natural as your own teeth. The first step is to see your prosthodontist to discuss treatments and find a solution to match your budget.

SIMONE'S STORY

Simone, age twenty-seven, came to see me six weeks before she was to get married. She had a tiny mouth, very asymmetrical lips, and an uneven smile: one side was up, the other down. She came requesting fillers to help augment and balance her lips. In evaluating Simone to understand how I could help, I started by asking her to smile. What I saw was dramatic. On one side of her mouth, the teeth were dramatically angled inward, while on the other side, the teeth almost stuck straight out. With some teeth practically crossed over and on top of each other, her mouth and lips were completely off balance.

I explained that the best approach would be to first address her teeth before I gave her any filler, because the filler wouldn't accomplish her goals without the proper support of her teeth behind her lips. She became tearful and explained she had just come from a visit with her dentist, who told her that she needed major jaw surgery, and then she would be required to wear braces for two years, followed by veneers. Thinking of myself as an honorary dentist after having attended so many of my husband's lectures, I suggested that she get a second opinion from him, hoping he would have a simpler and less expensive solution.

Six weeks later she came in for a follow-up appointment and for fillers, but she didn't need them because she looked magnificent! The difference in her smile was remarkable. It turned out that she had seen my husband as I suggested, and he had addressed the issue for her in just a few visits without surgery, using veneers to re-create her arch and bite. She loved her new teeth; they looked natural. She also noticed that her jaw felt better and even occasional headaches she had been experiencing were no longer a problem now that her bite was back in line. Her mouth and teeth also gave her a powerful boost of self-esteem, which sparked some deep soul-searching. She told me, "Once my teeth were fixed and I got my self-confidence back, I realized that my fiancé was not a kind man. I had put up with him only because my self-esteem was so low." She had decided to call off the wedding!

She remained a regular patient of mine, and two years later when she came into my office simply glowing, I said, "Oh my God, you have that glow that only comes from great sex and love—you look amazing!"

"I am in love!" Simone said. "I just got married to the greatest guy in the world." Her smile and her skin were beautiful, in large part because she was genuinely happy. That's the power of self-esteem. How you look and how you feel are inextricably connected. For this woman, fixing her teeth changed her life.

TREATMENTS

Treating the lips and perioral region is among the most delicate arts in the realm of facial rejuvenation, and easily done badly. Be sure to see a trained aesthetic physician. Depending on your age and the amount of sun damage and volume loss you have, a combination approach, using devices, fillers, skin care products, and chemical peels, is usually required. Neuromodulators can also be used to soften the movement that creates the lines, to treat a gummy smile, and to lift the corners of the mouth, but these are off-label uses and advanced techniques.

Fillers, ideally the HA (hyaluronic acid) fillers in the superficial category, help smooth the lines and enhance the lips. It is important to proceed slowly, with a doctor who understands balance and proportion, to make sure you look your best and don't end up with too much projection or that dreaded "duck lip" look. Treatment may take months, but beautiful results that will last for years are worth the wait. My favorite fillers for the lips are Restylane Silk, Volbella, Juvéderm Ultra, and Belotero. I sometimes layer these in and around the lips to create a lift-and-fill effect. The best approach to injection is to place the product more toward the center of the mouth to create a natural pout rather than a sausage lip. The dimensions are specific, unique to you, and can be measured at the time of treatment. It's most certainly an art, and we doctors must first understand the science of our tools to achieve beautiful results.

SKIN CARE

Retinol in its many forms is the most highly studied and published antiaging product in our medical literature. Creams with retinol or retinoids thicken the deeper collagen layers of the skin. This helps soften the creases and lines around the mouth. Over-the-counter products that contain alpha hydroxy acids also help to soften the appearance of lines around the mouth. For long-term results, your dermatologist can recommend specific products that also contain ingredients designed to naturally boost collagen, including peptides and growth factors.

Are You Afraid to Speak Your Mind?

Women have a long history of not saying what is on their mind for fear of hurting someone's feelings or seeming aggressive. We are taught to be "nice girls," putting our own needs after those of others and not speaking up. My namesake, actress Doris Day, challenged this notion in her Hollywood movie roles, which made her an exception in her time. She also famously said, "Age is just a number." I agree completely!

One of my most important roles as a physician and as a woman is to help my patients understand that it's okay and even feminine to speak up about how they feel or what they want, whether it's asking for equal pay or a promotion at work, or for their partner to participate more fully in the care of their home and family. It's so important to know that you have value and you deserve to be acknowledged, respected, and fulfilled in your life. That is true beauty!

ASK DR. DAY

The following are two of the most common questions I'm asked involving mouth concerns from patients and listeners of my Doctor Radio show on SiriusXM 110:

Q: *I've been battling severe perioral dermatitis [mouth rash] for a year now. I follow my dermatologist's instructions to the letter, but it comes right back. I'm an anxious person; could this be the reason it's recurring?*

DD: Actually, this condition is often a variant of rosacea (a skin condition characterized by facial redness, dilated blood vessels, papules, pustules, and swelling; see page 154). People often get bumpy and red skin in the middle portion of their face. Your dermatologist may treat your mouth rash similarly to rosacea on the face, with any single product or a combination of prescription medications like oral doxycycline; or topical gels or creams such as metronidazole, ivermectin (Soolantra), or azelaic acid (Finacea).

If you use teeth brighteners or whiteners, be careful to brush your teeth before you wash your face, because the chemicals for whitening and removing plaque can be irritating to the skin around the mouth and trigger a flare-up of perioral dermatitis.

There is also a medication called Oracea, which is often covered by insurance and can help control the problem. It's a low dose, time-released doxycycline that works as an anti-inflammatory without any antibiotic properties or issues of resistance, and can be very helpful for rosacea of the skin or eyes.

Q: *What are your favorite fixes for lines and wrinkles around the mouth?*

DD: I like to say your lips shouldn't touch unless you're kissing someone! One mindful thing you can do to smooth out these lines is to be aware of your expression: the less your lips touch, the softer those lines will become naturally. Practice keeping them slightly parted and watch those lines fade away!

The next step is to use serums and creams to help strengthen the skin and repair damage from repetitive motion. I love Restorsea LipMagic. Restorsea products use a special enzyme found in salmon eggs to target dead cells for exfoliation and rejuvenation of the lips. The process gives your lips a plumper look and more natural color. This can be combined with a prescription retinoid like Retin-A cream or an over-the-counter product containing retinol, which is to be used on the entire face including around the lips. Some of my other favorite products containing retinol are the Roc Retinol Night Cream, the Olay ProX Intensive Wrinkle Protocol, or Neutrogena Rapid Wrinkle Repair, which all have good science behind them and are in the $20-to-$30 range.

A more advanced level of treatment is fractional laser resurfacing. Be sure to allow seven to ten days recovery time. The fairer your skin, the more aggressive treatment can be. The nonlaser treatments that I like for the mouth area are eMatrix, EndyMed Intensif, and Pollogen Legend, which have less downtime and are administered in a series to stimulate collagen.

Another option your aesthetic physician may opt for, usually in combination with other treatments, is a neuromodulator like Botox Cosmetic, Dysport, or Xeomin very carefully placed to help smooth and evert the lips.

Fillers are also very helpful for these lines. The newest fillers, like Restylane Silk, Belotero, and Volbella, help smooth the lines and enhance the lips without adding bulk, so you don't end up with that duck lip look. As always, an aesthetic physician is your best resource for optimal results. For extra fullness, a more robust filler like Juvéderm Ultra XC or Restylane works very well.

Coming up...the most common complaint I hear, especially from my older patients, is about their chins and necks. The next chapter is devoted to this issue and includes exercises and a discussion on noninvasive treatments, as well as surgical procedures you can use to keep your chin up!

CHAPTER FIVE

Keep Your Chin Up—Tightening and Toning Your Neck

"We all look good for our age, except for our necks."

—*Nora Ephron*

When Nora Ephron turned sixty she realized that there was little she could do (on her own) to tighten and tone her neck. Thus, her hilarious book *I Feel Bad About My Neck* is devoted to musings about aging and other annoyances. Nora was right, of course. The neck ages faster and more poorly than the face, and it's an area we don't pay attention to until we don't like what we see. Patients tell me they apply sunscreen to their face but are not as good about applying or reapplying it to the neck or chest. The result over time is skin that looks like a plucked chicken—it's mottled red and brown with loose, sagging skin and cords from platysmal bands, which are muscles within the skin, and vertical necklace lines, without the necklace. There are also genetic conditions of excess fat under the chin, called submental fullness, and I will help you deal with these as well.

The simplest way to visualize the ideal of youth and beauty is to think of an "inverted triangle." In youth, the brows are lifted, there's fullness in the temple, the cheekbones are high, and the angle of the jawline is relatively sharp. The chin has a presence. Our focus goes toward the eye and the upper face or midface. As we age, we lose bone structure and fat and our chin recedes. This inverted triangle becomes a pyramid of age, and attention is now drawn to the lower face and neck. Minimally invasive aesthetic procedures are used toward the goal of restoring and maintaining a positive balance. We recover contour for the area under the chin and "reflate" (opposite of deflate) the face to recover volume where it's lost. This helps to recontour the face and neck so the area has a more natural, youthful appearance. Fortunately, to borrow a line from the musical *Wicked*, we now have ways of defying gravity.

"The good, of course, is always beautiful, and the beautiful never lacks proportion."

— Plato

THE PHI'S HAVE IT (OUR FACIAL STRUCTURE)

What the triangle of youth shows us, and what we see in art, is balance and harmony. Artists and researchers have actually calculated some of these ideal proportions and mathematically quantified this harmony. Arthur Swift, a board-certified plastic surgeon who teaches at McGill University in Canada, created the Golden Ratio theory, which is a mathematical relationship found in beautiful things (for you number crunchers out there, the ratio of Phi equals 1:1.618). You can see this mathematical Golden Ratio in architecture, music, and famous works of art, such as the sculpture *Venus de Milo*, a Stradivarius violin, and Notre-Dame Cathedral.

This same ratio can be applied to the human face. That said, if you're not Christie Brinkley or Angelina Jolie, it is nearly impossible to achieve this universal mathematical ideal. But what we can look for instead is balance. As the Smile Test on page 80 shows, when you look in the mirror, you will likely notice differences and imbalances when one side of your face is compared to the other. What you need to strive for is to create (or re-create) a facial balance and contour that is natural and makes sense for you as an individual. When this happens, you will end up looking more youthful. I truly believe that women in their fifties, sixties, seventies, and beyond can look even more beautiful with every decade.

Which brings me to that saggy area below our chin (also known as the submental region) that plays a key role in maintaining facial harmony and balance. One of the most common complaints I hear from my aging patients is about their double chin (submental fullness). According to an annual survey by the American Society for Dermatologic Surgery, 68 percent of people are bothered by the softening or heaviness of the neck and chin. The reason for this is that a sagging neck can make your face look unhealthy or fat, even if you're neither.

So what are some of the best ways to keep your chin up? Many of the procedures now available, such as focused ultrasound, which I describe below, along with fillers and neuromodulators, have had wonderful results in lifting sagging chins. Reflating the cheeks and redefining the jawline with dermal fillers can also lift the neck by adding discreet volume where it has been lost, literally lifting the neck and giving you natural, lasting results.

NONSURGICAL TREATMENTS

The following are the latest procedures to help you relieve that "pain" in the neck and help you get rid of that wattle. The results are beautiful!

Ultherapy

Ultherapy is an outstanding nonsurgical treatment for the face, neck, and décolletage that uses high-density focused ultrasound to lift and tone loose skin with no downtime. With focused ultrasound, we can actually lift and tighten the neck without cutting or disrupting the surface of the skin. Your body's natural response to the treatment is to replace tired and damaged collagen with new, stronger collagen, much like exercising builds muscle gradually and over time. Another plus is that the procedure requires only thirty to sixty minutes, and there is no special recuperation. Just one or two treatments can produce meaningful results, which can last for years. Ultherapy is also done in conjunction with other procedures, such as lasers and fillers.

Neuromodulators

These are off-label uses, but when administered by a trained aesthetic physician the use of neuromodulators can lead to smooth skin on the neck. While there is some risk of bruising, this treatment offers a very youthful appearance with no downtime otherwise. The first time I mention to my patients that I can treat the neck with neuromodulators, they are surprised and a little apprehensive, asking, "Will I be able to swallow?" The answer is yes, because I'm affecting the muscles within the skin of the neck and using doses that tighten without affecting the ability to swallow. The next time they come in for treatment, often before I've even fully entered the room, the first thing I hear is, "Don't forget my neck!"

If over treated, there can be side effects, including trouble swallowing, so it's very important to see an aesthetic physician who is trained to treat this area. Treatments need to be repeated at three- to five-month intervals for best results.

Fillers

Soft tissue fillers can also be used to fill in necklace lines and improve collagen and elasticity. The most common products used are Sculptra and the lighter of the HA fillers like Belotero and Restylane Silk while more robust fillers are used in the chin and along the jawline. This is also an area of advanced and off-label technique (meaning these are not areas specifically FDA-approved for these products), with the risk that the area can end up looking lumpy, so it is best to have the procedure done by a trained aesthetic physician. Improving the jawline and midface with fillers also helps rejuvenate and lift the neck. More robust fillers designed for mid or deeper layers of the skin are used in this case. Fillers also degrade at different rates in different parts of the face. The lower face tends to need more product and to need re-treatment more often than other areas such as the cheeks or midface.

Skin Care

Skin care for the neck always starts with sunscreen, sunscreen, sunscreen. There are excellent products available, and anything SPF 30 or higher will do. Beyond that, ingredients like retinol, growth factors, adaptogens, niacinamide, peptides, and vitamin C are excellent. You can use special firming creams that are specifically tested for the neck, an area that is often more sensitive than the face; or you can use your face products and extend them down your neck. My favorites are Revision Nectifirm, Senté Neck Firming Cream, and Neocutis MicroFirm.

Liposuction

Chin and neck liposuction will reduce excess fat in the jowls, under the chin, and on the neck. The doctor may combine traditional and laser liposuction to bring about the best results in both fat reduction and tissue tightening. The treatment can be done under local anesthesia. There is some downtime after the procedure, and sometimes drains are used for a day or so to minimize swelling. You will be required to wear a chin strap garment, so it's a good idea to take a few days to a week off from work. Before having this procedure, the doctor will evaluate whether you have enough elasticity in your skin to contract after the removal of the underlying fat.

Kybella

Kybella is an FDA-approved injectable that causes the destruction of fat cells to contour and improve the appearance of a double chin. The treatment is considered to be permanent, just as is the case with liposuction.

The product is made from a synthetic formulation of deoxycholic acid, a substance found naturally in the body that breaks down and absorbs dietary fat. When injected into the submental area, Kybella causes the fat to permanently dissolve, resulting in a more contoured and defined jawline. Most people will need from two to four treatments. Kybella may not be appropriate for patients with excessively loose skin. It works beautifully along with the above treatments to help rejuvenate the neck and take years off without surgery.

EndyMed Skin Tightening

EndyMed skin treatments can tighten the neck and lower jaw, as well as other parts of the body, including the thighs, abs, buttocks, upper arms, chest, and knees. EndyMed skin tightening uses deep dermal heating of collagen fibers to stimulate long-term tightening. Thermal energy targets the subdermal layer of the skin in order to stimulate the body's natural healing processes. Due to that stimulation, collagen begins to rebuild, leading to a tighter, firmer appearance in the treatment area.

Silhouette InstaLift

How many times have you sat in front of the mirror, pulled your skin along your jawline back toward your ears, and thought, *If only I could look like that again?* Well, an InstaLift treatment may be exactly what you're looking for. The product earned FDA clearance in April 2015. The sutures are made in the United States from a commonly used biomedical copolymer that is well tolerated by the body. The fully resorbable sutures lift and reposition the skin's subdermal tissue, while the resorbable bidirectional cones hold the sutures and facial skin in an elevated position. Over time, the implanted sutures and cones also stimulate collagen production to help increase and restore volume to the midface for natural-looking, long-lasting results. This procedure is becoming increasingly popular because it is done without surgery, and the lifting and sculpting effects are immediate with minimal risk and little downtime. There may be a slight transient skin puckering for a few hours to days after the treatment, and you can expect some tenderness for a few days to weeks afterward. This might be a good choice for those who notice a little sagging but are not ready for invasive surgery. It is also good for post–plastic surgery patients who want a little touch-up. However, it's important to be realistic about expectations associated with these quick-fix procedures. It is probably not an ideal choice for those who have a heavy chin, or those with thin, loose skin. This product works very well when used with neuromodulators and fillers.

Frequently Asked Questions

Q: *What are Silhouette InstaLift sutures made of?*
The sutures are made from poly lactic-co-glycolic acid (PLGA), a polymer that is frequently used in medical devices and is well tolerated by the body. The fully resorbable sutures have bidirectional cones that provide both lift and excellent anchoring of the subcutaneous tissue.

Q: *What areas of the face does InstaLift treat?*
The procedure lifts and helps increase volume and restore contours to the midface, cheek, and neck. It's also now being used on other parts of the face, such as the forehead, and the body as well.

Q: *Is general anesthesia required?*

No. Your physician will use only a local anesthetic to numb the area before inserting the sutures.

Posttreatment Tip: People Won't Notice What's Not There

When I was a teen and finally had my braces taken off after two and a half years of being a "metal mouth," I was so thrilled I went back to school eager to smile again to my friends. They asked why I had this silly smile on my face, but no one noticed that my braces were gone because they weren't supposed to be there. This is what I want for you.

People will notice that you look better, but they won't be able to pinpoint what has been done. If you are able to contour your submental fullness, people won't notice what is now gone. If we as cosmetic dermatologists do our jobs right, and you as patients don't have unrealistic expectations, people won't notice that you've had any work done because, like my braces, a heavy chin, or brown spots, or frown lines are not supposed to be there in the first place! You simply look better. So get ready for the compliments: "You look great! What did you do?" or "How come I know you for so long and you don't age?" or "How is it that you seem to be aging backward?"

Your Platysma Muscle

There are fifty-seven muscles throughout your face and neck that you probably never think about toning. Exercising the muscles in your face will make your jawbone more prominent, enhance your cheekbones, and help you shed that excess fat under your chin. The platysma muscle extends from the upper portion of the chest to the lower jaw and part of the face. This group of muscles, when toned, holds your neck and jawline upward in your youth but may separate during the normal aging process, leading to a drooping chin, sagging jawline, and turkey neck. By strengthening and toning your platysma muscle, you will help reduce the gobble, gobble for a younger-looking face.

CHIN UPS: NECK AND CHIN EXERCISES

Head and Shoulder Stretch

Doing simple daily stretching exercises for your neck will help keep your muscles flexible and toned. Tilting your head slowly from side to side or front to back will exercise the muscles of your lower face, jaw, and neck, engaging the platysma muscle group and creating a firmer jawline. Do these stretches, which have the added bonus of reducing tension that often congregates in the jaw and neck area, five to ten times several times a day, especially while you are sitting at your desk or computer.

Chin Lifts

This exercise will strengthen the platysma muscle, which is located in the front of the neck. Lie on your back, with your head hanging partially over the side of the bed. Place your hands at your sides, and slowly lift your chin toward your chest while exhaling. Hold your head up for three counts, then relax it back to its original position. Repeat this exercise three to five times per day. And this is yet another excellent area for off-label neuromodulator treatment. There are many women who get a dimpling of their chin when they speak, which is due to muscle movements of the mentalis, the main muscle of the chin. Botox Cosmetic in this area can not only smooth out the chin but also help lift the corners of the mouth. This treatment is an area of advanced technique, though, since there are many muscles, positioned very close to one another, that help you move your mouth in different directions. Therefore, your doctor needs to have a very clear understanding of anatomy and be very precise in the treatment in order to avoid distorting your smile or the movement of your lips when you speak.

Ceiling Kiss

As Annelise Hagen, author of *The Yoga Face: Eliminate Wrinkles with the Ultimate Natural Facelift*, explains, facial exercises such as the ceiling kiss can help keep the skin from sagging. Stand in front of a mirror, shoulders down, looking straight ahead. Tilt your chin toward the ceiling so you feel the stretch in the front of your neck. Now (I know this will sound strange, but trust me, it works), kiss the ceiling five times, pursing your lips upward and then relaxing. Turn your head to the left and do the same, then turn your head to the right and repeat. This facial yoga exercise should be done three times a day.

ASK DR. DAY

Q: *I'm sixty-eight, and my face is much more lax than it used to be when I was younger. I've had Restylane Lyft and Sculptra and I liked both of them, but I'm wondering which one will give me the most bang for my buck in treating skin laxity?*

DD: I use both of these products in the facial area and both are excellent options. Sculptra may last longer but it takes more treatments and you will get more immediate results from Restylane Lyft.

Q: *I'm fair skinned but blessed with looking younger than my chronological age. I'm fifty-five, though often people think I'm ten or fifteen years younger. I don't have wrinkling on my face, but I'm seeing some pouching on the side of my chin. Also, from my bottom* *lip to my chin I have a fold that is starting to bother me because it makes my upper lip look smaller. What do you suggest?*

DD: I always prefer to start with minimally invasive procedures. If you want to go further down the road, a lower face-lift can be an option. I would consider a three-pronged approach:

1. Neuromodulators like Botox Cosmetic or Dysport can help with the neck and the sagging at the corners of the mouth or jawline by tightening and affecting the balance in the area.
2. Tightening or lifting lasers and devices are excellent options, such as: Ultherapy, Thermage, EndyMed, Fotona, and even fractional resurfacing lasers that I use along the jawline. Sometimes a series of treatments is required for optimal results.
3. Filler placed properly and discreetly along the midface and jawline area can have the beautiful rejuvenating effect of a lift even if you have a turkey neck. One of the deeper fillers (see page 28) injected into the cheeks will lift them up. This is a great novel treatment that gives natural results for patients. And it can last up to two years, so it's more durable.

Remember, always look at the face as a global aesthetic, rather than focusing on a problem that bothers you. Treatment is about re-creating a youthful shape and obtaining balance and harmony. Your face has its own topography—with natural elevations and depressions.

Next, I will explain how to stop (or turn back) the hands of time!

CHAPTER SIX

Palm Reading

(How Are You Handling Your Life?)

"As you grow older you will discover that you have two hands;
one for helping yourself, the other for helping others."

—*Audrey Hepburn*

What do your hands say about you? Do they look and feel dry, chapped, itchy, or old? Those are important clues, and chances are the condition of your hands says much more than you realize. In this chapter I'll share with you what your hands can tell you about yourself, and I'll help you understand how you can better handle your skin and, of course, everything else too!

During a study, an observer was able to accurately guess the age of people by viewing only a photograph of their hands. This shows that our hands are a reliable indicator of how old we are, and sometimes they can even make us seem older than our years. Just as we take measures to retain a more youthful-looking face, we need to take care of our hands to help them look younger.

Let's start with Michelle's story. She's forty-two and came to see me about three months after giving birth to her first child—a beautiful, healthy baby boy. This is not just any baby; she had gone through six rounds of IVF to get pregnant, and she was determined to be the best mommy ever and take the best-ever care of the baby she had worked so hard to conceive.

Michelle complained of "horrible" rashes on her hands, which were red, raw, and cracked and thus itchy and painful. It didn't take me long to see that her hands looked like they had taken quite a beating, but I needed to know more before prescribing anything to help them heal. Upon further discussion, she told me how she was afraid to take her eyes off her son when he slept because she had read all about SIDS and she wanted to be there in case he stopped breathing. She also told me that she triple-washed her hands any time she touched "anything" in order to avoid spreading germs that could make her baby sick. The baby had quite a bit of colic, which she thought was caused by her breast milk, but she was told that breast-feeding was best for the baby, so she didn't want to stop. She was very careful about her diet, eating only organic, fresh foods that she prepared herself. She finally also confessed that she wasn't getting much sleep and that she was feeling depressed.

Her husband worked in finance and was often away on business trips, so Michelle was the main caretaker and didn't trust anyone else to help care for the baby. She was literally having trouble handling her situation, and it showed in her hands. I didn't need to know her well to be able to analyze her situation. Her body language and the extent of her rash told me the story. The details were unique to her, but the underlying message is one that is not uncommon, especially in moms of newborns and especially when it is the first child.

If you're a new mom, chances are you're washing your hands countless times a day: every time you change a diaper, prepare a bottle, pick up the baby, put the baby down—and the list goes on. Of course you don't want to make your baby sick or expose him or her to any germs, so you have to wash your hands again and again. This kind of anxiety can lead to telltale "mommy hands" like Michelle's. Although I have excellent products at my disposal to help heal the skin, in this case, they were more likely to simply mask the true problem.

I assured Michelle that she was not alone in feeling overwhelmed by the stress of caring for an infant. Having had two children, I know how wonderful but challenging being a mom can be. When I explained that it is impossible to wash all germs away from the skin, and that some exposure to germs in childhood actually helps develop the immune system and even prevent allergies and other immune-related diseases later in life, such as asthma, Michelle was able to relax. After taking my advice to find resources to help with the baby, and cutting down on the hand-washing (and hand-wringing), her problem with the skin on her hands disappeared for good!

When I was pregnant with my second child I had just finished my internship year at Bellevue Hospital, and I decided to spend a year working in a research lab at the NYU Langone Medical Center. It was a very exciting year of work, during which I studied the effects of retinol and certain vitamins on keratinocytes (skin cells) in culture. I learned so much, which to this day helps me in creating and evaluating skin care lines. However, part of the research involved tagging cells with radioactive material in order to follow the changes the cells went through in the experiments. This particular radioactive material doesn't penetrate beyond the outer layer of skin and I was always well-protected, but I was so anxious about any—even theoretical—risk of harm to my unborn child or to my toddler when I got home and hugged and played with her, that I washed my hands twenty to thirty times in a day. It didn't take long before I had skin that was raw, chapped, and extremely painful, just like Michelle's.

I spoke with my lab director, who explained how the skin of my hands offered the best protection against infection and even penetration of the radioactive material. By overwashing I was actually weakening my best defense. He explained that I was much better off simply wearing gloves, lessening the amount of hand-washing, and applying more moisturizer to my hands.

Within a week, my hands had improved and my anxiety level

was ten times lower. I trusted in my body to take care of itself, and I accepted the rational truth that my work was not hurting my baby. That was the first of many conflicts I've faced in maintaining a work-life balance. I realized that it wasn't just my hands; I was conflicted about being a mom with a full-time job. The tug-of-war between work and parenting is something many women have to face. The lessons I learned in the lab served me well and helped me to handle many situations that followed. I also learned that the work I do, which is part of my being fulfilled in life, made me a better wife and mother. My kids actually thrived as a result of growing up with a mother who was passionate and dedicated to her work, and we really valued the time we had together.

There are many examples of diagnoses where an acute rash tells a story, and we will discuss some of these in chapter 8: "Don't Be Rash." Regarding the hands, there are other changes that occur in that area over time that can give away your age as much as or more than changes in your face. Our hands often show the first signs of aging. Hands have little fat and few oil glands (the main source of natural moisture for the skin), and the skin is thinner than on other parts of the body, which is great as part of their overall design for mobility and flexibility, but not ideal for staying young and beautiful-looking. Hands that are mottled with puffy blue veins, brown spots, thin skin that reveals the tendons underneath, or short, cracked, brittle nails are like billboards advertising that you've reached a certain age. Even with regular application, it's hard to keep moisturizer or sunscreen on the hands because of how much we wash and use them—they take quite a beating over the course of even a day, let alone years.

This was the case for my patient Charlotte, in her mid-fifties with five grown children, when she came to my office to show me her hands. She is an executive assistant and balances a busy life between work and family. I examined the back of her hands and noticed immediately that the right and the left looked like they belonged to two different people. One was smooth, while the other had brown spots, large veins, and thin, translucent skin. "Do you play golf?" I asked her. "Yes, how did you know?" she said, looking surprised. Although I didn't know much about the sport, I told her I did know that golfers often wear a glove on one hand, so it was obvious which hand fell victim to sun damage. She played only on the weekends, which speaks to the scourge of ultraviolet rays. Still, golf had been her passion since college, and the years of exposure had taken their toll on her skin (Beyond Beautiful lesson: it's never too early to care for your skin!). I wouldn't have dreamed of telling her to give up the sport, because doing what you love helps keep you young in mind, body, and spirit, but I did suggest that she wear sunscreen on both hands and reapply every two hours. I was happy to learn that she wore a visor, but I recommended one that was wide-brimmed and that she use a generous amount of sunscreen with SPF 50-plus as well.

If you spend time outdoors, taking some simple protective measures can prevent age-related damage to your hands. If you wash your hands after using the bathroom or before eating, reapply the sunscreen (I never leave the house without my powder sunscreen in my purse). My favorite sunscreen powders are from ColoreScience and ISDIN.

ASK DR. DAY

Q: *I read that the FDA has banned soaps containing triclosan. Are antibacterial soaps and hand sanitizers with other ingredients a safer choice? Also, how long should I wash my hands to make sure they are disinfected?*

DD: As of September 2017, the FDA ban will include eighteen chemicals in addition to triclosan that are contained in soaps. This chemical is also found in wipes and even some cutting boards in our desire to be as germ-free as possible. Antibacterial sanitizers eventually morphed into a whopping $1 billion industry. More than forty years of FDA research—along with countless independent studies—have shown no evidence that triclosan provides any health benefits compared to old-fashioned soap. Equally concerning is that antibacterial soaps have the potential to create antibiotic-resistant bacteria. If you are on the go, use an alcohol-based hand sanitizer instead.

As for how long to wash, rub your hands together under warm (not superhot) water until you work up a good lather, and don't stop until you finish two choruses of "Happy Birthday." (This is a good way to teach children how long they should wash before meals.)

GETTING A HANDLE ON YOUR HANDS

Here are some common hand conditions that I treat, followed by tips to help you turn back the hands of time.

Problem: Prominent Veins, Translucent Skin Revealing Underlying Tendons

Lost volume and ropy veins and tendons that pop out of your skin can make your hands look old and craggy. Like sagging necks, this is something that inevitably occurs over time, but fortunately there are outstanding nonsurgical, minimally invasive treatments available.

Problem: Liver Spots or Age Spots

Liver spots, also called "age spots," get their name from the fact that they are the color of liver and they occur with age, not because they have anything to do with the health or function of the liver. They typically develop in people with a fair complexion, but they can also develop on darker skin.

Liver Spots or Age Spots

- are flat, oval areas of increased pigmentation;

- are usually tan, brown, or black;

- occur on skin that has had the most sun exposure over the years, such as the backs of hands, but can also appear on the tops of feet, and on the face, shoulders, and upper torso;

- range from freckle size to more than half an inch (thirteen millimeters) across and can group together, making them appear more prominent.

TREATMENT OPTIONS

Fat Grafting

Fat grafting involves the transfer of fat into the hands from donor sites such as the knees, thighs, love handles, and tummy, which decreases the visibility of bones, tendons, and veins on the back of the hand. Not much fat is needed for this procedure, but it can be costly—to the tune of $10,000 or more—and requires anesthesia for the fat removal. Several treatments may be needed for lasting results. Because of the level of effort and skill required, many people opt for fillers instead.

Fillers

Injectables such as Radiesse are an excellent option for restoring a youthful appearance to the hands, and the results last a year or longer. Clinical trials are under way using Voluma and other hyaluronic acid fillers for this purpose as well. The amount of filler required for each hand depends on several factors, including the amount of volume loss and the patient's individual goals. There is usually some amount of tenderness and swelling after injections with a dermal filler, but it normally recedes in a few days to two weeks. Fillers take very little time compared to fat transfer and are also a fraction of the cost.

Topical Treatments

To give your hands some extra TLC, make sure you moisturize them every time you wash. Trade in your traditional antibacterial hand sanitizer for a combination sanitizer that contains moisturizer or lotion and use it only if you're on the go. Cetaphil Gentle Skin Cleanser and Aveeno Ultra-Calming Foaming Cleanser are good for both the hands and the face. Skin often becomes extra dry during cold-weather months, so look for rich, creamy moisturizers (without fragrance) during the winter and know that the best time to apply them is right after the bath or shower.

The more sunscreen you use on your hands from an early age, the less likely you are to get that translucent skin, not to mention sun spots.

Go Coconuts

Coconut oil is a prime example of an ingredient that is better for you when put on your body than when put in your body. As a food, it's higher in saturated fat than even butter, and studies show it causes an increase in the bad LDL cholesterol. However, as a topical, it has antibacterial and antifungal properties, can fill in as a natural moisturizer for dry hands, and smells delicious! It's great for soothing your dishwashing-parched digits, so keep a jar by your kitchen sink. You can get coconut oil at your local grocery or health food store. You can go with straight-up organic extra-virgin coconut oil, or mix your own handmade moisturizer consisting of coconut, shea, and jojoba butters. Coconut oil is great for your hair, too, which I will discuss in chapter 7. And, alternatively, another one of my favorites for these uses is sunflower oil.

Gimme Some Sugar Scrub Massage

A sugar scrub can do wonders in making your hands look and feel soft and smooth. I suggest using this in the evening when you are finished with your chores and ready to relax. Simply mix enough sugar with a nonfragrant, plant-based oil to make a pasty scrub. Now massage your hands with the mixture and leave it on for five minutes. Shut down your devices, turn off your TV, and take a few minutes to close your eyes and breathe during the wait time. Rinse off with lukewarm water and apply a moisturizer when done.

Handle with Care

As a dermatologist who is personally and professionally involved in the testing of skin care products, I came up with my own line called Esteem, which you can order from my website www.myclearskin.com. One of my products, Handle with Care, is formulated with natural extracts (including coconut, of course) that decrease inflammation enzymes to soothe the skin, remove irritation, and reduce redness while repairing the skin's barrier function for increased hydration. Just look at some of the ingredients in this cream, which you will want to get your hands on: cactus extract, coconut fruit extract, coconut ester, vitamin E, and panthenol (provitamin B_5).

ASK DR. DAY

Q: *I recently turned sixty-five, and I've begun to notice a number of unsightly brown spots on the backs of my hands. Some are larger than others and some are in clusters. Should I see a dermatologist to check if any of these spots are skin cancer or are these just age spots?*

DD: You should have a dermatologist evaluate your spots, especially if they are dark or have changed in appearance, to make sure they don't need further attention or biopsy to rule out a skin cancer. Your doctor may also offer several treatment options alone or in combination:

LASER TREATMENTS

More good news. Many treatments that work for your face will also work for your hands. For those of you in your thirties, I suggest starting early with preventive options, such as light peels and laser treatments. These include intense Fraxel 1927 and Fotona, which target brown sun spots. The zapped spots will eventually dry up and fall off. Voilà!

Recovery can take one to two weeks, and home care is very important to help speed up recovery and minimize the need for further treatment. The main factor to consider when having laser treatment is the amount of energy used and the skill of the doctor. The skin of the hands and body react very differently than facial skin. The face heals better and can handle more energy than anywhere else on the body. It's not intuitive, but it's true.

CHEMICAL PEELS

There are excellent chemical peels using phytic, glycolic, and other acids along with ingredients to minimize redness that can help even skin tone and stimulate rejuvenation. Depending on the peel, there may be less downtime than with laser treatment, but peels also require more sessions and may not be as effective as a laser.

MY TIPS FOR HOME CARE

Light and Bright Cream

Another product from my Esteem line is Light and Bright Cream, which reduces and removes the appearance of age spots on the hands and arms. It features a new, proprietary EpH quinone technology, an innovative biomimetic whitening complex that inhibits melanin production.

Out, Out, Damned Spot!

Hydroquinone is the gold standard for diminishing brown spots, but it can be irritating to the skin. Other less potent options include kojic acid, alpha-arbutin, licorice extract, and vitamin C. You can try combining two or more to get an extra bang for your buck. If you want a ready-to-wear OTC product, try Dr. Lewinn Kinerase Skin Tone Perfecting Serum XK, which contains kojic acid and licorice extract.

Lighten Up

For hands mottled by sun damage or hormonal conditions (like melasma), spot treatments might not do the trick. They can create a halo effect with areas of lightness on a dark background. For an all-over treatment to combat sun damage, try a brightener like Kiehl's Photo-Age Corrector Intensive Corrective Moisturizer with vitamin C, either by itself or combined with a spot treatment.

A lightening product that also contains a chemical exfoliator like glycolic or salicylic acid can help erase age spots by gently sloughing off dead cells, which brightens the skin. Vichy ProEven Dark Spot Corrector with exfoliating salicylic acid and vitamin C is available at some CVS stores. SkinMedica Lytera 2.0 is also an excellent hydroquinone-free brightener that does not contain retinol, which makes it more tolerable for sensitive areas like the hands. Retinol can be used separately as needed.

Retinol Rescue

You know what a fan I am of retinol for all kinds of skin care. It also improves skin tone. If you see brown spots starting to form, a retinol cream can keep them from getting darker. To improve texture and lighten dark spots, apply retinol at night and an alpha hydroxy cream with sunscreen during the day on the back of your hands. Don't forget to apply the broad-spectrum sunscreen daily; otherwise, the spots will return, no matter what fading treatment you use.

Glove It or Sleeve It

If you spend a lot of time in the sun, like my patient Charlotte does on the fairway, or if you are driving during the day with the sun streaming through the car window, gloves will protect your hands, and long sleeves will cover your exposed arms to prevent sun damage. Sun protective clothing works even better than sunscreen, so learn to glove it or sleeve it!

HAND EXERCISES

According to the National Center for Biotechnology Information in Bethesda, Maryland, those ugly enlarged veins on your hands might lead to carpal tunnel syndrome, the condition that usually comes with repetitive movement of the fingers as when using the keyboard (or texting on smartphones). Certain hand exercises can help reduce the appearance of prominent veins and ease the tenderness and nerve pressure that sometimes accompany them. Exercises like the ones below work by pumping the muscles and stimulating blood flow to help drain accumulated blood away from the engorged veins.

Hand and Finger Stretch

Reach your arm out in front of you and bend back your fingers with your other hand to stretch out the wrist and fingers. Next, do each finger one by one. Repeat the stretches on the other hand. Then gently bend the thumb forward and back inside your hand and outside your wrist. Do this exercise at least once a day.

The Boxer

Stretch your fingers out as wide as you can, then clench them into a tight fist. Repeat five times.

The Prayer

Place your hands together in a prayer position at the center of your chest and push together. Then raise your elbows out to your sides while dropping your wrists down toward your belly button. This will give your wrists a good stretch.

ASK DR. DAY

Q: *I'm fifty-nine and I'm interested in plumping up my hands. Can you suggest any options?*

DD: People typically lose volume in their hands with aging, and this causes the veins and tendons to be more visible. To help replace the lost volume, I like to use fillers such as Radiesse, which is FDA-approved for hand augmentation and rejuvenation and is one of my favorites. Some doctors use Voluma or other hyaluronic acid fillers to plump up the hands, while others do fat transfer, but the latter is more involved and also more expensive. I recommend having several treatments over four to six weeks, rather than one session, in order to minimize side effects and optimize results.

My hands have always been thin, and when I hit about forty, I felt that my hands were looking older than the rest of me, and certainly older than I felt. So I had my own hands treated, and I absolutely love the results. They're still thin and I can still see the veins, but I don't mind that because the quality of the skin is so much better and my hands feel soft and smooth. I love my hands!

NAIL IT!

When you look at your hands, what do you see? Maybe you notice that you need to trim, clean, or stop biting your fingernails. No big whoop, right? But if you ask a dermatologist, she or he can see a whole lot more. Your nails, like your skin, tell your dermatologist a great deal about your health, including factors ranging from poor diet and stress to potentially serious problems such as kidney or liver disease.

The most common problem I see, however, is weak or splitting nails. This tells me that patients are not getting proper nutrition, water, exercise, or enough sleep. When someone comes to see me, I always pay attention to their hands and especially the nails. If your cuticles are ragged, and your nails have been bitten to the nub, I know that you are worried or maybe just have too much stress in your life and need to do some soul-searching or mindful Beyond Beautiful techniques (see chapter 9).

This was the case for Kelly, a patient in her late twenties who, other than her hands, was an attractive young woman. As I was talking to her I watched her pick, push, and bite at the cuticles around her thumbnails. I asked about her life at the moment and she volunteered that she was under a lot of stress at work. She was very distressed that her boss was taking credit for some of her important achievements. Kelly was aware that she was biting and picking at her nails, which can be a form of obsessive-compulsive disorder (OCD) and cause a habit tic deformity that permanently scars the nail, but the action was very comforting and nearly impossible to stop once started. The resulting nail changes look like a series of irregular indentations going up the middle of the nail from the cuticle all the way to the tip. I encouraged her to see a therapist to talk about her anxiety and problems at work and explained that her nail problem might be related to a condition such as OCD, assuring her that this was not her fault and that the right balance of medication, if needed, along with cognitive or talk therapy, would not only improve her nails but also positively impact her work and happiness.

In the meantime, I recommended that she get a monthly manicure. Most include a hand massage—heavenly—a pedicure to give her pretty toenails, and a leg massage to boot! She took my advice and came back for her next visit with prettier nails, and the smile on her face told me that her self-esteem had already gotten a big boost.

As you've learned by now, having healthier, better-looking skin and nails depends on the inextricable connection between our mind, body, and skin. That's why I encourage you to give yourself an instant lift starting right now by taking good care of your nails. The following is some info that will help you nail it!

NAIL CARE AT YOUR FINGERTIPS

Nails consist of the nail plate, which is the part you see; the cuticle, the tissue that covers the base of the plate; the nail bed, the skin beneath the plate; the nail folds, the skin that supports the nail on all three sides; the lunula, which is the "half-moon" shaped section seen at the base of the plate; and the matrix, which is under the cuticle. It is usually most visible on the thumb and index fingernails.

I know someone is a nail biter if I see the lunula at the base of all the fingernails; it's a sign of stress of the nail and the nail trying to recover from the insult, in this case, from biting. There are also some medical conditions of the liver and the kidneys that affect the color of the nails and the lunula, which is one good reason why it's so important to see a dermatologist if you have any concerns about or see unwanted changes in your nails.

Nails are made of a type of keratin, the protein that also makes up skin and hair (this is why many shampoos and conditioners contain keratin). Fingernails grow faster than toenails, and the rate of growth is affected by such factors as age, gender, and even the season. Nails usually grow faster when you're young, if you're male, and if it's summertime. The nails on your dominant hand grow faster than those on the other hand. Nails will also grow faster if you are in good overall health.

ASK DR. DAY

Q: *My cuticles are a wreck. I know I'm not supposed to cut them, but what else can I do to fix them?*

DD: Think of your cuticles as your friends. They serve an important role in protecting your growing nails from damage and infection. If you look closely at your thumbnail or index fingernail (without nail polish on it), you will see a small white semicircle just above the cuticle. This area, called the lunula, is where nail cells are made. As the nail cells grow, they are pushed outward and eventually reach the tips of our fingers, where we eventually cut or file them. The area of the lunula also extends and sometimes is entirely contained in the area under the cuticle. Damage to the area of the lunula, by either trauma or infection, can lead to scarring, followed by permanent deformity of the nail. When you pick at your cuticles, you are potentially traumatizing the lunula as well as increasing the risk of infection. For this reason, your dermatologist will recommend that you either leave the cuticle intact or just have the manicurist gently push it back without removing it. While nail polish can be a little drying to the cuticle, it is really the drying effect of the acetone in the nail polish remover that does most of the damage to both the cuticle and the nail. Be sure to rinse off and moisturize after using nail polish remover. It also helps to wear gloves when doing dishes or any work where your hands will be in water for more than a few minutes. And, of course, be sure to moisturize every time you wash your hands (and, of course, moisturize your hands, not just your cuticles, but do pay attention to the cuticles when you moisturize).

THINNING NAILS

People who don't eat well and have vitamin or dietary deficiencies may have thinner-than-normal nails, which are more likely to break. If you have weak nails, some nail-strengthening foods to introduce in your diet include salmon (wild-caught), which is high in vitamin D (good for bone growth) and vitamin B_{12}, a deficiency that can cause nails to become dry and darkened. Salmon is also an excellent source of anti-inflammatory omega-3 fatty acids, which are good for our skin and just about everything else.

Eggs also contain vitamin B_{12}, vitamins A and E, iron, and biotin (a part of the B-complex vitamins, also known as vitamin B_7 or vitamin H). Biotin has been scientifically shown to increase fingernail thickness and reduce brittleness and splitting.* Plus, the protein in eggs, unlike meats, is highly digestible and easily absorbed by the body.

Beans, which are rich in biotin, are another good nutritional choice for those with thinning nails. In one Swiss study, participants with brittle nails were given 2.5 mg of biotin daily for six months. Amazingly, the participants' nail thickness increased by a full 25 percent. Almost any bean is nutrient-packed, but lima beans are especially rich in calcium, magnesium, zinc, copper, potassium, phosphorus, vitamin K, and no less than six B-complex vitamins. You can read more about Beyond Beautiful nutrition in chapter 9 (page 192).

BEAU'S LINES

Horizontal lines on the nails, also known as Beau's lines, are often associated with serious physical stress. Appearing as an indented line across the nail, they frequently occur in people who have gone through chemotherapy. Beau's lines also occur after some illnesses, injuries, or with severe malnourishment. There may be an altitude connection too. They've also shown up on the nails of scuba divers who dived 1,000 feet and on the nails of those who climbed Everest. If you are not undergoing chemo treatments, scuba diving, or climbing high mountains, see your doctor for help to get rid of unwanted Beau's lines. Vertical nail lines, however, are different. Some people are more genetically prone to them than others, and they're commonly associated with natural aging and dryness of the nails.

---

* V. E. Colombo et al., "Treatment of Brittle Fingernails and Onychoschizia with Biotin: Scanning Electron Microscopy," pt. 1, *Journal of the American Academy of Dermatology* 23, no. 6 (December 1990): 1127–32, http://www.ncbi.nlm.nih.gov/pubmed/2273113.

FIVE REASONS YOUR NAILS MIGHT BE FAILING YOU

If your nails aren't looking so great and you wouldn't dream of telling someone to "talk to the hand," here are five possible causes (and solutions) you can point to (if you're brave enough).

1. Nutrient Deficiencies

Nutritional deficiencies such as anemia and vitamin D and protein deficiencies, as well as changes in other organs, such as the liver, kidneys, and heart, can all show in the nails. We may see spoon nails, especially in cases of an iron deficiency; dark or light nail bands, in patients with liver issues; or half-and-half nails, where the white area of the nail is excessive, in the case of kidney issues. A study published in the *Journal of Cosmetic Dermatology* found that taking 2.5 mg of vitamin B daily improved nail strength and reduced brittleness after six to nine months. While protein deficiency is rare, if your nails are peeling at the tips or showing ridges (both signs of brittleness), biotin might help. Vitamin D deficiency also affects the nails. Solution: Ask your doctor if it would be appropriate for you to take a 2.5 mg dose of biotin once a day, along with a vitamin D supplement, to reduce brittleness. I highly recommend getting vitamin D from food or supplements rather than from exposure to the sun. It might take several months to see results, and, as always, you should talk to your doctor before you take any new drug or supplement. Also, be aware that skin cancers, such as melanoma, can also occur in the nails, so any nail changes should be brought to the attention of your dermatologist for evaluation.

2. Lack of Moisture

As I wrote earlier, it is important to reapply hand lotion (and sunscreen) every time you wash your hands. Water dries out your skin, and if your cuticles are also dry, the underlying nail matrix will feel like a desert, too, and your nail will be prone to splitting, breaking, and cracking, and may develop longitudinal ridging. Solution: Find a fast-absorbing lotion like CeraVe Therapeutic Hand Cream or Neutrogena Norwegian Formula Hand Cream, or even simple coconut or olive oil, and apply it throughout the day. Don't forget the area above the matrix from the cuticle to the second knuckle of your finger.

3. It's All About the Base and the Top Coat

I know you thought it was manicure 101 to never skip the base coat, but guess what? You were wrong. By putting a base coat directly on nude nails, the chemicals in acetates can eventually eat away at the plate, making it weaker and more likely to break. Solution: The first step in your manicure process should be applying a small amount of hand lotion to your nails before polishing. The lotion acts as a primer, filling in the tiny gaps in the nails while hydrating them so they're not at risk of damage from the base coat and polish. Wait for the moisturizer to dry, wipe away any excess, and polish as usual. The top coat can help hold moisture in the nail and help discourage overdrying of the nail when you wash your hands.

4. You're a Cuticle Picker

Some people are cuticle crazy, so back away from the cuticle cutters and just say "no" if your manicurist asks if you want them cut. These bits of skin at the base of the nail are essentially a bodyguard between your nail and skin, shielding your nail from water, bacteria, and anything else you touch. Cutting the cuticle removes that safeguard, which leaves nothing to prevent water or other things from entering and causing an infection. Solution: Tame your cuticles by gently pushing them back with a washcloth after you shower—no cutting allowed, ever!

5. *Your Polish Remover Is Like a Chemical Spill for Your Nails*

If you take a whiff of your polish remover, you won't be shocked to learn these nail strippers aren't exactly born in nature. Acetone in traditional remover strips the natural oils in your nails along with the polish, leaving them brittle. Unfortunately, even non-acetone removers can be drying. Solution: Look for a soy-based, acetone-free option, such as Priti NYC Soy Nail Polish Remover, which contains oils that leave nails moisturized not neutralized.

———

Next…if you've noticed changes in your hair, I'll explain what that means and what you can do to prevent or treat it. I'll also explain how to get rid of unwanted hair, the best products to use to protect your luscious locks, and salon secrets for coloring, treating, and styling aging hair.

CHAPTER SEVEN

The Hair-Raising Truths and Treatments

"I'd love to kiss ya, but I just washed my hair."

—*Bette Davis*

Hair is not just an accessory; it's powerfully tied to our self-esteem, confidence, and sense of beauty. When your hair looks thick, full, beautiful, and sexy, everything in life is better. I see women every day who complain of hair thinning and loss. Some of these women are as young as in their teens or early twenties, while others are in their fifties and beyond. They are of all different ages, but they have similar fears: fears of going bald, fears of losing their beauty, fears of how they will look tomorrow. So many of these women come to me greatly frustrated because they have seen doctor after doctor and are told there is nothing wrong and that they have plenty of hair. They are told that it's all in their head, or that it's all stress-related, so they should relax; or, even worse, they're told there's very little they can do about it—it's just genetics. Hair thinning and loss is one of the most difficult, complicated, and frustrating issues for a dermatologist to address as well. From the doctor's perspective, the office visit usually plays out like this: The patient comes in for any reason other than hair loss. Then, at the end of the visit, just as the doctor is ready to walk out the door to see the next patient, thinking she's covered everything, the patient mentions, "Oh, and I also have hair loss." This happens for several reasons, the main one being that most people are embarrassed about hair loss and feel so helpless that it takes a lot to bring it up even with their doctor. The other major reason is that they feel hopeless because they've already seen doctors about their hair loss concerns to no avail. They are looking for validation and to be taken seriously. They are often desperate for a treatment and sometimes even nearly suicidal over the amount of hair they see coming out on a daily basis.

A whopping thirty million American women experience hair thinning and hair loss by the time they're fifty. After many years of studying the research on the causes and treatments, as well as observing and treating patients with hair loss, I've learned that there are confluent medical and emotional drivers of hair thinning. Our hair, like our skin, gives us many clues about our overall health and well-being. What hair issues tell me about a patient is very specific and consistent with the way the patient is managing their life and their stress. Here's a recent example: I saw a beautiful Indian woman with long, thick, silky hair. When I walked into the exam room, she was already tearful and immediately told me she was there because of ongoing issues with hair loss. I examined her scalp and could, in fact, see areas of thinning as well as many short hairs of the same length, which were a sign of hair regrowth. I could also see that she did not have a genetic pattern of hair loss, an autoimmune issue involving the hair, or scarring of the scalp that would imply any other underlying medical issue. I ran through in my mind the differential diagnoses of possibilities, and the long-term outlook did not match her level of concern or distress. I needed to know more to be able to help her. Upon further discussion, I learned that she was a lawyer working her way up to partner, and she was committed to her work and her goals, and thus working very long hours. She also told me she had recently become engaged, and that while the meeting of her potential future husband was arranged, she had choices and was very happy about the engagement and looking forward to the marriage. The wedding would take place back home in India in six months. Everything sounded rosy—too rosy. I investigated further: "Do you have any siblings or does he?" "Yes, and they are so much trouble," she told me. "His sisters hate me, and his mother wants me to stop working once we get married. She is putting pressure on her son and is stressing the relationship." She also shared that her work was very busy and she didn't have all the time both families needed and demanded of her because she was working on so many cases at once. Nowhere in this conversation did I hear anything about what she wanted or what would make her happy. It was all about pleasing everyone else. She was literally being pulled in too many directions— at work being overloaded with cases, at home being asked to manage opposing forces, and with friends who were against even the idea of a marriage that was in any way arranged. She wanted to please and appease everyone around her, and she wanted to do a great job with everything she did. I could practically see her hair shedding as she spoke. This wasn't simply a case of increased stress; this was a very specific type of anxiety, and it didn't surprise me at all that she was experiencing hair loss. I was able to help her with products for hair loss; and, by shining a light on the true underlying cause, she was able to have a great wedding and move up the ladder to become a partner at work.

The facts are astounding: in the United States alone, eighty million people are affected by hair loss, and over 50 percent of all women will experience some form of hair loss in their lifetime. Every day I see women who are deeply depressed, sometimes to the point of feeling suicidal over the thought of going bald. Hair is not just a simple, irrelevant appendage or accessory. It is strongly tied to our self-confidence. A head of thick, healthy, flowing hair can make us feel gorgeous. This is why more than $2 billion is spent each year in trying to avoid or reverse the effects of hair loss and thinning.

A fifty-two-year-old woman who had thinning hair in the temple and crown region came to my office with her husband. A wife and mother who worked full-time, she told me her hair was coming out in handfuls. She also had some issues with arthritis. She had gone to her primary physician for blood tests to see what might be causing this hair loss, but the test results were all normal. I examined her and saw that when the light hit her at a certain angle you could see her scalp, which was understandably extremely upsetting to her. She told me that she was no longer able to change her hairstyle enough to hide her bald patches, which made her feel too uncomfortable to go out with her husband. She also confessed that she spoke incessantly about her hair with her husband and constantly asked him if he noticed how bad it had gotten, until ultimately their conversations were all about her hair. It got to the point where they stopped having sex because she was feeling less attractive. She felt that her husband was angry at her about this and that her life was spiraling out of control.

There are commonalities in the two cases I just described, and the same is true for the vast majority of those who are preoccupied with hair and hair loss, whether or not they have a genetic or hormonal pattern. It's not by accident that hair loss is your issue instead of an ulcer or acne or other conditions. There is so much I can help you with in managing the hair loss and it's important to treat it, but it's equally important to take note of the driver of the issue and to heal from within in order to help the treatments work and to live a better, more fulfilled life. Rather than just putting a Band-Aid on the problem, this is true healing, what I call Beyond Beautiful.

For the Beyond Beautiful connection, try this quiz:

Hair Loss Personality Quiz

Are the following statements true or false for you?

You are ambitious.	True/False
You are a pleaser.	True/False
You have a hard time saying "no."	True/False
You have a lot going on between work, friends, and family.	True /False
You feel overloaded.	True/False
You feel torn between all the different factions of your world.	True/False

If you answered "true" to three or more of these questions, stressors in your life may be accelerating your hair shedding, thinning, and loss. Identify what you truly have control over in your life and what you can do to alleviate some of the pressure you feel. The commonality I see in patients experiencing hair loss, whether or not there is a genetic tendency, is this: they are bright and ambitious, and they are high achievers who have a lot going on at once. They also like to be in control, to have "every hair in place," figuratively if not also literally. They are often pleasers who take on more than they can handle, and they don't know how to say "no." The Beyond Beautiful lesson here is to learn to be more self-centered. This is different from being selfish. Being self-centered means understanding that you are responsible for your own happiness and well-being, not for the happiness and well-being of others; it means learning to say "no," politely but firmly, and letting others manage more for themselves. By taking responsibility for your joy and well-being (and by letting others take responsibility for theirs), your odds of stopping your hair thinning and loss greatly increase. It's very liberating and will work wonders for your hair.

BRUSH UP ON HAIR LOSS FACTS

Despite a wealth of information we now have about beauty, aesthetics, and treatments for women of every age and ethnicity, I still see hair loss as an issue that is misunderstood. There is no "silver bullet" solution for hair loss, which remains a highly emotional, embarrassing, and private concern for many women. Numerous celebrities wear wigs or extensions that make it appear as though they have tremendous amounts of hair, and this sets a high bar for the person who has an average amount of hair. Hair commercials appear every day on TV and in magazines, featuring beautiful actresses and models touting hair treatments and shampoos that supposedly give voluminous, thick, silky, smooth hair. Late-night infomercials advertise hair loss treatments using lasers, products, and transplants, all promising the moon to an extremely vulnerable audience.

Given these unrealistic expectations, it's important to be armed with some basic facts. These include understanding the difference between predictable changes in hair and true hair loss, and knowing what to expect from the time of your first appointment through diagnosis and treatment.

WHAT TO EXPECT FROM YOUR DOCTOR'S VISIT

Getting to the root cause of hair loss (the medical term is alopecia) generally involves a physical exam, sometimes with blood work, and possibly a biopsy of the scalp before an official diagnosis can be made. Here's what to expect when you visit your doctor:

Dermatologists will start with a general exam of the skin on your scalp. They will examine your scalp with a lighted magnifier looking for redness, scaling, irritation, and scarring of the skin as clues to any condition that might be affecting hair growth. They will also notice any obvious patterns or patches of hair loss.

In examining the hair they will look for even the most subtle changes or shifts in your hairline, spotting recession at the temples, increased spacing between the hairs, and patchy sections of thinner hair. In some cases, a gentle pull test may be required. Don't worry, it doesn't hurt!

Don't be surprised if your dermatologist also examines your face and other parts of your body to check for other areas of visible follicular hair loss, scarring, acne, and hirsutism (excessive and unwanted abnormal hair growth) or any correlation of other conditions affecting additional parts of the skin and body that might also be causing or contributing to the hair loss.

Sometimes the diagnosis is followed with a series of blood tests to check essential hormone, thyroid, and vitamin levels. In some instances scalp biopsies will also be recommended if the dermatologist is concerned about scarring or a medical condition causing the hair loss.

THE FOUR MOST COMMON TYPES OF HAIR LOSS

Once a physical exam and blood workup are complete, a dermatologist will be able to assess the core (or collective) factors that are related to your hair loss type and cause.

1. Hereditary (Androgenetic Alopecia)

For 95 percent of men and women, the diagnosis will be hereditary hair loss (officially called androgenetic alopecia). This can begin to present even in the early twenties, and for women starts with a slow widening of your hair part, the result of thinning in the crown region (at the top of the scalp). Unlike men, you won't notice any recession in your frontal hairline.

2. Stress Shedding (Telogen Effluvium)

If you experience a major life event, positive or negative, such as childbirth, the death of a loved one, marriage, divorce, or illness, about three months after that event you may notice that your hair starts to dramatically shed. The reason for the lag is due to the changing hair growth cycles. The medical name for this condition is telogen effluvium, and it's one of the most common diagnoses a dermatologist makes when it comes to hair. It can take up to a year for the cycles to rebalance, but the hair that sheds in these cases is growing back, even if it's hard to tell in the short term. Constant stress often leads to recurring telogen effluvium or stress shedding and can also accelerate the natural aging of your hair. If you are shedding, it's the hair that's falling out, not the follicles themselves. The follicles are there and have the capacity to regrow and do regrow over time.

3. Traction Alopecia

This is a scarring hair loss that results from years of traction caused by things like tight braids, extensions, or any process that adds excess pull and weight on the hair. Though years may pass before it occurs, once it does, the follicles are lost and the hair will not regrow. Therefore, it is important to minimize trauma caused by pulling on the hair or overprocessing as much as possible. Newer hairpieces are much lighter and gentler on the scalp and help reduce the risk of traction. They are temporary and have to be used on a daily basis, but they are preferable to hair extensions for the reasons just stated.

4. Immune-Related

Immune-related hair loss, such as alopecia areata, occurs when the immune system mistakenly attacks the hair follicles. The cause of the immune trigger remains a mystery, but telltale signs are visible clumps that have fallen out, creating completely smooth, round hairless patches on the scalp. In some cases the loss can progress to all the hair on the scalp and face, which is called alopecia totalis; or to the hair on the entire body, which is called alopecia universalis.

The Modified Hair Wash Test

This is a noninvasive test underutilized by dermatologists due to a lack of familiarity with the test. It is very helpful in distinguishing between chronic telogen effluvium and androgenetic (hereditary) alopecia. You can do this test at home.

1. Avoid washing your hair for 5 days before the test date.
2. On the day of the test, cover the sink with gauze.
3. Shampoo the hair thoroughly and rinse.
4. The hairs trapped in the gauze are collected, counted, and divided into hairs less than 3 cm and more than 5 cm long.

Results:

1. If 10 percent or more of the hairs are 3 cm or shorter and if there are fewer than 100 hairs total, that is a sign of androgenetic or hereditary hair loss.
2. If fewer than 10 percent of hairs are 3 cm or shorter and there are more than 100 hairs total, that is a sign of chronic telogen effluvium.
3. If more than 10 percent are 3 cm or shorter and there are more than 100 hairs shed, that is a sign of having both conditions simultaneously.
4 Finally, if fewer than 10 percent are 3 cm or shorter and there are fewer than 100 hairs shed, that is a sign of chronic telogen effluvium that is in recovery.

"Although my hair loss was completely widespread across my entire body, Dr. Day was convinced we could find a miracle."

Madeline Gross, who came to me with alopecia universalis (total hair loss), shared her story on my Facebook page. It has a happy ending, and I give it a million "likes"!

"I was diagnosed with alopecia universalis during my freshman year of college and, just when you think you're entering the best four years of your life, everything begins to change. After five years of hair loss and bouncing around from dermatologist to dermatologist, I finally found Dr. Day, who was never going to give up no matter what it took.

"Although my hair loss was completely widespread across my entire body, Dr. Day was convinced we could find a miracle. I saw her continuously for two years every six weeks for cortisone injections, and although the pain was unbearable she constantly gave me breaks to check on me and make sure we could continue with the procedure. Although this disease is very hard to track and there is no cure, Dr. Day convinced me to never give up and to always have a positive outlook on the rest of my health.

"Recently we stopped the cortisone shots and began an oral drug, and after just a year on the prescription I now have a full head of hair, eyebrows, eyelashes, and the most dreaded...leg hair!!! In six years, I have never felt more like myself than I do now, and I have no one else to thank besides Dr. Day and her team. No matter if I was walking into their office with drawn-on eyebrows and a wig or with a ponytail and long eyelashes, they always welcomed me with open arms and made me feel very comfortable!! Love you guys!"

HAIR TREATMENTS

If you are suffering from hair loss, know that you are not alone, and be sure to see your dermatologist to learn of the newest and most promising treatments. The good news is that this is an area of very active research, and recent advances have given hope for long-lasting cures in the near future. Sometimes a combination of procedures, products, and medications shows the best results, which is why you must work closely with your doctor to find what's right for you. The following are the latest high-, medium-, and low-maintenance treatments available at this writing:

Minoxidil

As the active ingredient in Rogaine, minoxidil is proven to help stimulate hair growth in both men and women. Over-the-counter options are available in up to a 5 percent concentration, but your physician can prescribe higher strengths and formulas that add in other ingredients to improve absorption and efficacy based on your need. Don't forget, this is a lifelong commitment to daily use! No exceptions, I'm afraid. The good news is, it keeps working as long as you use it. If you ever do decide to stop, it won't make more hair fall out; rather, you'll simply revert back to where you would have been if you had never used it. Most things we do for health and rejuvenation need to be done indefinitely, and hair growth is no exception.

Supplements

Nutrition also has an impact on your hair, and for healthy hair you need to make sure you're getting adequate levels of the right vitamins (especially B and D), and a proper balance of proteins and healthy fats. This makes the difference between a full, thick shiny head of hair and thin, brittle dull hair that sheds and breaks easily. Some supplements that I have seen excellent results with include:

Nutrafol is a high-performing cocktail of ingredients and adaptogens including bioactive keratin, curcumin, vitamin D, ashwagandha, and other ingredients, with data showing support in hair health and growth.

Viviscal contains AminoMar, vitamins C and E, silica, hyaluronic acid, and collagen.

Low-Level Light Therapy (LLLT)

There are several in-office laser devices as well as at-home devices that are FDA-approved for hair growth. Since there are several brands and types, be sure to ask your dermatologist which one is best for you before investing in a device for home use.

Platelet-Rich Plasma (PRP)

You might have heard about this treatment being used on the face and joints, but while not FDA-approved as of yet, it has also been shown to be an effective hair regrowth treatment. The dermatologist will take a small amount of your own blood and spin it down to separate out the pure platelet-rich plasma, which is then injected into the scalp to stimulate regrowth by harnessing the power of your body's own stem cells and growth factors. Yes, science is amazing!

Hair Transplantation

We've come a long way since the days of unsightly hair plugs. New techniques that use follicular unit extractions and robotics create natural-looking hair transplant grafts that restore fullness and balance to thinning areas, grow to be long and strong, and create a beautiful hairline. This is another procedure in which technique is critical, so it is very important to see a hair transplant expert. Women who have good donor hair (i.e., areas, usually at the back of your scalp, with hair that is strong and healthy) have found this to be a very effective treatment. Outstanding advancements in robotic surgery have helped to optimize the process by minimizing scarring and improving graft success.

Hormonal Balance

Even just slight shifts in your hormone levels can wreak havoc on your hair. The prescription drug spironolactone, which is not a hormone, may be prescribed off-label to help offset hormonal imbalances, depending on the pattern and severity of your hair loss. It is also used for acne and unwanted hair growth on other parts of the body. Some doctors prescribe finasteride and other medications more commonly used by men; these medications have not been approved for women. Be sure to see a dermatologist who specializes in hair if you are considering any of these medications.

JAK Inhibitors

There has been active research on a new class of drugs, called JAK inhibitors, that have been shown to be promising in the treatment of autoimmune forms of hair loss, such as alopecia areata and alopecia universalis, and, possibly, hereditary hair loss as well. This could be a game changer for those suffering from these conditions, so ask your doctor if you might be a candidate.

DIY Hair Mask

Setup and ingredients:

Mixing bowl
Whisk or large spoon
Shower cap
2 to 4 egg yolks (short hair needs 2; medium needs 3; and 4 for long hair)
3 tbsp. castor oil
1 tbsp. coconut oil
1 tbsp. dark organic honey
2 drops rosemary oil (helps mask the scent of the castor oil)

Mix the ingredients in a mixing bowl with a whisk or a large spoon. Apply the mixture to damp hair from the scalp to the ends. If your hair is long, twist it into a loose bun at the top of the scalp. Place a shower cap over the hair and leave on for 15 to 30 minutes.

Lather with your regular shampoo and then rinse with warm water. It's important to add the shampoo before the water in order to effectively remove the oils without leaving the hair greasy. Rinse again with cool water. Dry and style your hair as usual.

ASK DR. DAY

Q: *I've always had oily skin and scalp, and my hair is thinning on top. After shampooing my hair, four hours later it's greasy again. My scalp is also itchy, but I don't have that much dandruff, although I use Head & Shoulders shampoo with selenium sulfide in it.*

DD: The problem of having a greasy, oily scalp is not uncommon. Believe it or not, Botox is FDA-approved to treat excess sweating, called hyperhidrosis, of the underarm, but it can also work on the scalp when injected directly into the areas of concern. It works by helping to block the contraction of the tiny muscles that squeeze sweat out of the glands. Other treatments you should consider trying first: Leave the dandruff shampoo on long enough to do its job. Try applying the shampoo directly to the scalp about five minutes before you go into the shower. You might also try a salicylic acid preparation, which will better penetrate the follicles to help the top layer of the skin shed off faster and more efficiently. Look for shampoos with 2 or 3 percent salicylic acid, like Neutrogena T/Sal Therapeutic Shampoo. There are also prescription products your dermatologist can recommend for you.

INTERVIEW WITH JULIEN FAREL,
Chairman and Founder of Julien Farel Haircare
with Anti-Aging Balance Technology

Q: *Please explain what happens to our hair as we age.*

JF: I've been obsessed with hair problems since I was fourteen years old. Let's start with the bad news. The hair ages the same way the skin does. When the skin ages it loses collagen and hydration. The same thing happens to our hair. On the skin, when you age you wrinkle. On the hair, you lose color, thickness, and strength. You might start with dry hair that eventually leads to hair loss. Hydration is everything. That's why we have products that penetrate into the scalp to keep the follicles hydrated. Without it, your hair will become lifeless.

Q: *What do you suggest for women with hair loss?*

JF: At my company we have used the advanced technology of the skin and applied it to the hair to produce an anti-aging hair product called Restore, which works like a miracle. It all starts with the scalp. Hair is like a flower. It will start dying first from the root. We use six proprietary compounds, including peptides and essential fatty acids, that contain everything the hair needs to preserve it. I also suggest using a serum at night, which is when the cells work to repair damage. When you wash your hair you use shampoo, which likely contains sulfates that produce a lather. People wash their hair with products that strip the hair of its hydration. After you shampoo, your hair can age ten years. Restore has no sulfates or parabens or detergents, so you won't see suds, and it will help restore and repair the hair, starting from the root.

Q: What are your recommendations for hair color and length as we get older?

JF: You must use a color that is right for your skin tone and eye color. If you can't afford to go to a professional, try starting with a hair color that is two shades lighter than what you see on the box because the formulation will be darker than you think.

As for length, I refuse to say that all older women should have short hair. Some younger women look great with short hair and some older women look great with longer hair. It's more important to select a style that works with the shape of your face and bone structure. Having the right color and hairstyle will give you more confidence!

Q: Is it okay to go gray?

JF: It depends on what kind of gray you have. Gray hair comes from the loss of melanin. If your hair is completely white, your hair can look great. The problem with going all gray for people with light complexions is that white on white skin can make you look like you are sick. Some people have a beautiful shade of gray and can look fantastic. Others can look like they aged fifteen years in one day.

Q: How often should we wash our hair?

JF: It's okay to wash once a day, but if you want to shower again after working out, just rinse off the sweat and apply conditioner to the ends only. At the end of the day you want your hair to smell good. Be careful not to use too much conditioner. If you have greasy hair, you need to wash your hair daily because you don't want the oil in the hair to damage the follicles. Oily-haired people should only put conditioner on the roots and not on the scalp. Use a good shampoo that doesn't contain detergent that will strip your hair. Hydration of the hair is the most important. Make sure your conditioner does not contain too much silicone.

Q: Is it okay to brush your hair when it's wet?
JF: You can brush or comb your hair when it's wet. I suggest brushing or combing your hair while you are in the shower to make sure that all of the product is out of your hair. Your hands can't reach all your hair, and you don't want to leave shampoo behind after you rinse. Brushing is good for the hair. It's like massaging the scalp. Both circulate the blood, which makes the hair look healthy. Start from the ends and work up to the roots. Make sure to use the right brush and don't pull on the hair, work through any knots or tangles very gently, and know that it helps to brush your hair before going in the shower to work through the knots before you wash. Brushing wet hair can increase stress on the hair, so start with a wide-tooth comb to loosen any tangles before going to a brush. Towel drying is fine.

Q: Will hot combs or blow-dryers damage the hair?
JF: Apply a balm on the hair when using a blow-dryer or hot comb to help protect against the heat. Put it on the roots and comb it through. Your hair can help to make you look pretty, but you must take care of it. Don't pass the blow-dryer or comb over the same area too many times—if you get a lot of flyaways, it may be a sign that you've overdried your hair.

DR. DAY'S RECOMMENDED HAIR PRODUCTS

I recommend the following products, which are safe for your hair and, in some cases, produce hair growth. Check Amazon or the company's website for current pricing.

Esteem Hair Growth System

Dr. Day's three-step system for hair regrowth consists of a specially formulated shampoo and conditioner that work together to prepare the scalp for the Rapid Growth Serum. Visible results can be seen within thirty days of use.

1. **Replenish Shampoo.** Replenish Shampoo removes daily product and scalp buildup and rinses clean, leaving the hair with healthy body, volume, and shine. Gentle enough for everyday use, Replenish creates thicker, fuller-looking hair, cleanses and fortifies the scalp, and stimulates hair growth while combating hair loss.

2. **Esteem Conditioner.** This panthenol-rich formula conditions and adds fullness to thin, lifeless hair by expanding the shaft of individual hair follicles, protecting and nourishing healthy hair growth, which creates the effect of thicker, healthier-looking hair.

3. **Esteem Rapid Growth Serum**. My Esteem medical-grade formula contains a biomimetic peptide, combined with a red clover extract rich in Biochanin A, to prevent hair loss and slow thinning, and to stimulate new hair growth (www.myclearskin.com/products).

Julien Farel Vitamin Restore

Julien Farel Vitamin Restore is an antiaging hair treatment that uses a fusion of potent revitalizing ingredients, including hydrochloric acids, and sophisticated skin care technology to reactivate the hair's life force, giving it optimal health and youthfulness. Applied directly to the scalp, Vitamin Restore is a nonfoaming hair treatment that cleanses, treats, and conditions hair in a single, simple step. It prolongs color brilliance and is ideal for hair that is weakened by stress, overprocessing, environmental damage, or seasonal changes. Restore is free of sodium lauryl sulfates (SLSs) and parabens, and no product testing is done on animals. For best results, use it every other wash (www.julienfarel.com).

Julien Farel Magnifique Fortifying Serum

This remarkable antiaging hair serum is formulated with cutting-edge bioactives that delay the graying process. Magnifique stimulates the pigmentation process by boosting melanin levels to slow the graying of hair and restore the hair's youthful texture and appearance. Ingredients include echinacea, edelweiss stem cell extracts, and hyaluronic acid to deeply hydrate layers of the scalp and hair. Magnifique is ideal for the treatment of hair thinning or hair weakened by stress, overprocessing, environmental damage, or seasonal change and is SLS- and paraben-free. This serum is designed to be used once a week or, for more intensive treatment, two to three times a week for three months when experiencing hair loss or during seasonal changes. It won't make your hair or sheets greasy. Julien Farel says if you use this product regularly, you won't have to get your hair colored so often (www.julienfarel.com).

Kirkland Signature Moisture Shampoo

The Kirkland Signature Moisture Shampoo, which is the Costco brand, is made of pure organic extracts. It's safe for all types of hair and has a moisture nutrient complex that promotes thick, healthy hair. Some customers say they stopped using a conditioner after using this product.

It's a 10 Miracle Volumizing Shampoo

This lightweight, sulfate-free shampoo is designed to remove daily buildup while also nourishing and strengthening hair. It's ideal for delicate, fine, thinning, or pixie-short hair. The hero ingredient is *Althaea officinalis* (marshmallow) root extract, which helps give lift, body, volume, and lightweight conditioning with absolutely zero residue or heaviness. This hair nutrition in a bottle also works to improve your hair's health by reducing scalp irritation and dryness—imparting even more weightless volume. Other ingredients include acai extract for strength and shine, soothing chamomile extract, green tea extract, and sunflower seed extract, a natural "sunscreen" that guards against dryness and color fading or brassiness. Learn more at itsa10haircare.com.

HAIR REMOVAL

The opposite of hair loss problems is having unsightly facial hair, which can make us feel masculine or like the bearded ladies that used to be at carnivals. Excessive hair growth on a woman's face can indicate an underlying medical condition involving the pituitary gland, adrenal gland, or ovaries. If you have coarse hair on your upper lip or chin, bring this up with your doctor. The majority of women, however, have some facial hair, more like peach fuzz, on the cheeks, or a light mustache after puberty, and at least a few annoying coarse chin whiskers after menopause. This is not a cause for concern but should be evaluated to rule out any hormonal or other medical issues.

DIY methods that might work for you include tweezing, shaving, or over-the-counter depilatories. The problem with these is that they need to be repeated regularly, even daily, and they may irritate the skin and create redness or stubble, and you don't want to kiss your spouse or partner with a scratchy face—even if you have to deal with a man's five o'clock shadow. I know a lot of women who swear by waxing, but I don't get it. How do you let your hair grow long enough to wax it off? That's just not attractive. I also see patients who have issues with ingrown hairs afterward, and this seems to be more of a problem with waxing than with other forms of hair removal. Another method that has lasting results is electrolysis. Although it's considered permanent, most people require maintenance treatments after electrolysis, sometimes for years, until all the hair stops growing back. It works by damaging hair follicles with tiny jolts of electricity and should be done by a certified practitioner. There is some risk of discoloration or scarring, and people with sensitive skin may find it painful unless a topical anesthetic is used prior to the treatment.

Shaving is an excellent option. I like the multiple-blade Venus by Gillette. With this and other razors with multiple blades, you typically need to pass the razor over the area only once, which helps avoid irritation or ingrown hair that often comes from passing the blades over the same area many times.

The best hair removal method, in my opinion, is laser treatments performed by or under the supervision of a dermatologist. I use a diode laser, which is the gold standard and can treat a broad range of skin types. Like electrolysis, it is considered permanent, but maintenance touch-up treatments may be needed every few years. And the best part is, the newer devices use special technology that makes them fast and virtually painless. The entire underarm and bikini areas can be treated in just a few minutes; legs and back take about fifteen minutes each. Unlike with waxing, it is important to shave before the treatment. The treatments are done at one-month intervals. Most people need six to eight treatments. Avoid hot showers for a day or so after the treatment and wear loose clothing so you don't rub against the treated area.

Whatever method you decide to use to get rid of unwanted hair, I guarantee that it will make you feel better about yourself, especially when you wake up in the morning with smooth, hairless skin!

PFB Shaving Cream

For a great, close shave, try my PFB Shaving Cream. It's rich cream, not a foam or lather. It stays down at the hair roots to give a clean, smooth shave that feels better and lasts longer than those given by traditional shaving creams.

Next...smooth, flawless skin is what we all strive for. It defines beauty and ensures confidence. Unfortunately, nearly everyone breaks out at some point or another during their lifetime, whether it's with acne, hives, poison ivy, or rosacea. This creates a barrier between our beauty within and our ability to put our best face forward. The good news is, as you will learn in the next chapter, if treated early and properly, rashes and pimples can be controlled and, ideally, completely erased!

CHAPTER EIGHT

Don't Be Rash—Breaking Out Isn't Hard to Cure

"I had just started ninth grade when I got my acne. And I had braces. I wouldn't look people in the eye. It was not a good time for me—it just killed my self-esteem. I thought when I didn't look at someone, they couldn't see me."

—*Kendall Jenner, supermodel*

It's never by accident that you break out in acne or a rash where you do and when you do. As my dear friend Dr. Jane Greer helped me see, if you don't understand the Beyond Beautiful connection, you will miss the opportunity to learn the important message your body is conveying. You absolutely still need proper medical attention to treat the rash or condition, but true healing and longer-lasting results come when you understand and also address the entire cause of the rash, which often goes much beyond the skin.

That was the case for Selma, a patient I regularly saw in clinic while I was a medical resident at NewYork-Presbyterian Hospital/Weill Cornell Medical Center. She had psoriasis that was relatively well-controlled with prescription skin creams, and every four to six months she would come in for a checkup and refills. Out of nowhere she suddenly had a severe flare-up of psoriasis to the point where it covered her entire body leaving her red and covered in scale (the medical term for this is erythroderma). When this happens, the body can't effectively regulate water balance or temperature and also has increased risk of infection, any of which can be life-threatening. She was hospitalized and treated and thankfully fully recovered to the point where she was able to return to her usual daily routine. About a year later the same thing happened. When I went in to examine her, I reviewed her chart history and noticed that at literally the same month nearly every year she would have a severe flare-up of her psoriasis. I found this very odd. Was it the change of season or some other identifying factor that would cause a potentially life-threatening intensification of her psoriasis at the same time every year?

Her chart did not reveal any sort of explanation, so I sat down with her to see if she could help me understand. When I explained to her that I could see a clear pattern of a flare-up at the same time every year and asked if anything happened at about that time that could account for this, she became really quiet at first and I could see tears welling up in her eyes. This caught me by surprise. I never expected to hear what she told me next.

She told me the story of her son, her only son, who was an honors student and had won a scholarship to a prestigious college. As a single mom, her son was her everything. She was very proud of him and how he focused on his studies, never did drugs, and did not let himself get pulled into the gangs that so riddled their neighborhood. He was in his last semester of college when one day, ten years ago to the month, he was riding on the subway and was shot during a gang-related shooting. He was an innocent bystander, the only one shot, and the only one not involved with the gangs. She said she wished her life could have ended with his, or better, instead of his. She felt she had failed him and she didn't feel she had the right or desire to go on living when he was gone. He had been her everything, and now she had nothing. Every day was a struggle, but the month of his passing was unbearable. Even now, ten years later, the memories were as painful as the day it happened. She said I was the first to notice the connection; she hadn't even made it herself because she had so deeply suppressed the feelings, and understanding the association was really powerful for her.

I made sure that the proper multidisciplinary team became involved in her care, including grief counselors who helped her to connect with support groups and other methods to handle her pain. The following year I suggested we try something different. I asked her to come in to see me once a month for a few months before the anniversary of her son's death, and I asked her to bring in pictures of her son on those visits so we could celebrate his memory together. She also told me of the support group she was now leading for mothers who had lost their children. She hadn't been ready to do that before, but now she was at the point where she felt strong enough to share her grief with others and to help others avoid the added complications to their grief that she had experienced. She avoided having a flare that year and, gradually, her psoriasis improved and she needed only annual follow-ups to review her care.

PSORIASIS

Psoriasis is an autoimmune condition with a genetic basis. The skin in the affected areas acts as if it has been wounded and creates new skin cells, which develop and turn over at an inappropriate rate—every four days instead of the normal month or so it takes for healthy skin. This turnover happens so quickly that the cells don't even have time to mature and slough off as they should, creating thick, red, itchy unsightly plaques. The most common areas we see this include the elbows, knees, and scalp, but it can happen anywhere you have skin, including the palms of your hands, the soles of your feet, and even the genitals.

The more friction or trauma you have in the areas, the more the condition is triggered, which is called the Koebner response. As with any condition, stress can be a trigger and managing stress along with overall health has an impact on this skin condition even more than others because psoriasis is pro-inflammatory and can affect other organs as well, especially the joints, leading to a destructive arthritis. Every patient with psoriasis needs to have regular visits with their internist and sometimes also with a multidisciplinary team that includes rheumatologists and cardiologists to make sure any signs of internal involvement are addressed as early as possible.

Treatments

There are exciting new treatments called biologics that can help control psoriasis as well as psoriatic arthritis or other internal manifestations of the condition. Your dermatologist will help you determine whether light treatment, a topical, or a biologic is right for you. Diet alone has not been shown to cure or fully control psoriasis, but a healthy diet will help any other treatments you choose to work better.

ACNE

Acne is the most common skin disorder in the United States, affecting more than seventeen million people. It's a myth that acne occurs only in teens; in fact, it can be a debilitating, scarring, disfiguring condition that anyone at any age, and of any gender or ethnicity can suffer from. Acne oftentimes doesn't begin until age twenty or older. We spend billions on creams and treatments for acne, and there is very active research looking for a cure. I'm proud to be part of the Acne Cure Alliance, created by Ray Chambers and devoted to ending the scourge of acne and the scarring that often goes with it. The distribution of acne on the face tells a story. I've also written a book titled *100 Questions & Answers About Acne* that dives deep into the underlying causes of and treatments for this common condition. Teen acne is usually found on the central face and forehead, while adult acne is more common in women and usually appears along the lower face and neck.

Stressed Out, Break Out

It is important to understand the impact of acne, which is more than what you see on the surface because acne is not simply a rite of passage of the teen years, nor is it "just" a skin condition that may be unsightly but will pass in time. Acne, even if it's mild, can lead to scarring and can have a powerful impact on a person's self-esteem. Even if you get only one new pimple a month, if that one pimple leaves a scar, that's twelve new scars a year. Over time, that adds up. And now that I've been in practice for twenty years, I've seen those who had mild acne scarring in their teens and twenties hit their thirties and forties and display something I had not read about in any textbook or medical journal or heard discussed at any meetings I attended: The mild, barely visible acne scarring of youth became deeper and more obvious with age. The collagen and elastin in the skin had deteriorated from years of sun exposure, and genetic aging exposed the bound-down unhealthy collagen of the acne scars.

Although stress does not directly cause acne, it does exacerbate it. Where the acne shows up on your face and body also tells a story. For example, when I see a teenage pattern of acne in an adult I know there's something more going on. An example of this was described by a caller to my radio show: Judy called in asking for advice about her daughter Julia's acne. She told me her daughter had mild acne as a teen, treated by her local dermatologist with excellent results, but now it was back and was leaving scars and ruining her daughter's beautiful skin. Nothing seemed to help. She explained how she was on her daughter's case, telling her to use medications regularly, not to pick, and to avoid eating chocolate and greasy food, but her daughter wouldn't listen. She said she was frustrated for her daughter and was trying to do everything she could to help her.

I was taken by how involved the mom was with her adult daughter's acne. Thinking this was a straightforward case of adult pattern hormonal acne I asked if the distribution was along the lower face and jawline, expecting to hear I was spot-on. Instead, I was surprised to hear that it was over the entire face—including the forehead and cheeks. This pattern was more consistent with teen acne.

This required further investigation. There was much more to the story: It turned out that while Julia was in her second year of college, she became pregnant. The relationship with her boyfriend ended, but she chose to have the baby and ended up transferring to a college closer to home so her mother could help care for her child, help her to make ends meet, and help make it possible for her to continue her education.

I asked the mom how much she liked having her daughter home, and she said she "loved" it. I asked her how much her daughter liked being home, and she said she "hated" it. I could hear from the mom's voice that she was still very much the "mom" and her daughter, now a mother herself, was still being treated as the "child." It was as if Julia were regressing back to being a teenager, even as she herself was raising her own child. No wonder her acne was acting up! Julia was conflicted, and her skin was sending her a strong message.

Once I explained to Judy how this acne pattern was telling an important story, she could see what she needed to do next and how she could be more helpful and supportive to her daughter, whom she clearly loved very much. I could hear the relief in her voice. We spoke of treatment options such as blue light and Isolaz, along with topical retinoids, benzoyl peroxide, and supplements that contain niacinamide. Julia's mom now had powerful information to help her daughter in a meaningful and lasting way, and she helped herself too. I also explained that acne isn't caused by eating greasy food, but it does respond better to a diet high in antioxidants and low in simple sugars and the avoidance of processed foods when possible.

There are many over-the-counter, in-office, and prescription treatments available. Here are some of my favorites:

Topical and Oral Prescription Medications

Your dermatologist can recommend a prescription treatment plan to help clear your acne quicker, and this often can be used along with over-the-counter and in-office treatments. The following topical treatments are usually used in various combinations, depending on the severity of acne and the sensitivity of your skin.

Benzoyl Peroxide (BP)

This treatment comes in wipes, gels, creams, foams, and washes of various strengths. There are both over-the-counter and prescription versions available. I prefer lower concentrations of 5 percent or less, since they work well and are less drying and irritating than higher concentrations. Also, be aware that this ingredient can bleach fabric, so be careful what your skin touches until it dries. For this reason I usually recommend it as a wash for the body.

Salicylic Acid

This is available over-the-counter at 0.5–2 percent strength in a wash, lotion, or other formulations and can offer eight- to twelve-hour shine control. These products have become more sophisticated over the years and have contributed to the arena of acne treatments. Neutrogena Naturals Acne Foaming Scrub has 1 percent salicylic acid, which helps cleanse, exfoliate, and control oil.

Oils for Acne

For the longest time oil and acne didn't mix and everything for acne had to be labeled "oil-free" to be believed effective, even though the science proved otherwise. Now there are over-the-counter oils used to help treat and control acne symptoms. Some of these contain coconut oil, as in the Skinfix Foaming Oil Cleanser, which is free from harsh sulfates, parabens, phthalates, synthetic fragrances, silicones, soy, gluten, and dairy.

Oral Antibiotics

The most common ones used for acne are various formulations of minocycline or doxycycline. There are new formulations that are better absorbed and can be used in lower doses, which has helped greatly in reducing the side effects of stomach upset and yeast infections in women. You should use a topical benzoyl peroxide if you're taking an oral antibiotic, to help reduce the antibiotic resistance of the *P. acnes* or other bacteria causing the acne flare.

Topical Antibiotics

These include topical clindamycin and topical erythromycin, sometimes used in combination with benzoyl peroxide to improve efficacy and reduce antibiotic resistance. Newer formulations are in the works for topical minocycline as well.

Retinoic Acid, Retinoids, Tazarotene, and Adapalene

These are natural or synthetic variants or derivatives of vitamin A and are the most highly studied and published ingredients for the treatment of acne. A bonus is that they also help the skin look young and radiant. There are so many formulations available, both over-the-counter and prescribed by your dermatologist, that I can safely say there is a retinoid out there for everyone—and anyone who can tolerate one should be using it. Start as a teen, and stay on it for life for beautiful, healthy skin. You do need to use sunscreen, since you will have increased sun sensitivity.

Topical Dapsone

This is available by prescription as Aczone, a topical 7.5 percent gel, designed to be used once a day to treat all the different types of acne: blackheads, whiteheads, papules, and pustules. I like to prescribe dapsone in combination with other topicals and orals. It does not make you more sensitive to the sun, and it does not contain benzoyl peroxide.

Hormonal Contraceptives (the Pill)

The synthetic hormones found in some oral contraceptives can decrease the secretion of oil from your glands, which can actually lessen breakouts. The ingredients in birth control pills vary, so you should work with your doctor to ensure that your medication contains the right mix of hormones. Some are better for acne than others. I prefer YazB, Estrostep, and Ortho Tri-Cyclen. One brand I usually avoid prescribing is Loestrin.

Oral Isotretinoin

Previously available as Accutane but now available only in generic forms, this drug is reserved for the treatment of severe scarring acne or acne that has not responded to other medications. It is highly effective, but a patient needs to have a thorough discussion with the dermatologist before taking. The common side effects are dryness of the skin, eyes, and mouth. But the more serious side effects are catastrophic birth defects if you get pregnant while taking or within a month after, and the risk of depression and suicide. I have seen outstanding results with Accutane, and I hope we never lose access to it, but it must be used with caution and under the tight supervision of a dermatologist.

Chemical Peels

These are a popular way to treat acne and to minimize scarring. Several different solutions are available for peels, and each has its advantages and disadvantages, so talk to your doctor about which one is right for your skin. Types of peels include glycolic, salicylic acid, Jessner's solution, trichloroacetic acid, and a new actinage peel, which is extremely effective in clearing the pores and producing fresh new skin. Some have more downtime or peeling; these should not be administered if you have a suntan and should be done with caution if you have skin of color.

Microdermabrasion

This procedure involves blasting fine crystals at the skin, then vacuuming them back up to clean out pores and exfoliate the skin. These treatments are a popular option that can improve skin texture, clear blackheads and whiteheads, and even out surface discoloration.

Lasers and Devices

I don't recommend lasers for active acne; however, the pulsed dye laser targets the redness and can speed up clearance of marks left behind as the acne clears. Isolaz is a device I often recommend for active acne treatments. It uses a photopneumatic process to loosen and extract blackheads, excess oil, and other contents from deep within your pores, immediately followed by a specialized wavelength of intense pulsed light delivered to your skin that helps to destroy acne-causing bacteria and to reduce redness and inflammation. These treatments are often used in combination with prescription medications to speed up and improve results. The Fotona laser also produces excellent results in the treatment of active acne, helping it clear and minimizing redness, discoloration, and scarring.

Cortisone Injections

This is a mainstay of in-office acne treatments. A tiny needle is used to inject the steroid right into the pimple or cyst. It is a safe treatment that localizes the medication right on the trouble spot, but there is a slight risk of localized thinning of the skin, which is usually concentration-dependent and often resolves within a few weeks to months. The treatment works best when done early on in the inflammatory process to both minimize the inflammation and clear the lesion faster.

Blue Light Therapy

Using a blue light with or without a photosensitizing agent called aminolevlulinic acid (ALA) can have a powerful impact in treating acne. This needs to be done with caution if the ALA is used because it takes about twenty-four hours for the ALA effect to wear off, and the skin will be extremely light-sensitive during that time. It's great for back and buttock acne since those areas are easy to keep covered after the treatment, but treatments on the face should be done with caution during the summer.

Treatment of Acne Scars

Even mild acne can leave behind discoloration and scarring, which is a change in texture of the skin. I have learned to treat scarring in my patients when they're younger and when the skin has the greatest ability for repair, if possible, to avoid having deeper and harder-to-treat scars as they age.

Soft Tissue Fillers

Bellafill is FDA-approved as a safe and effective dermal filler. It is frequently used to treat acne scars and pores by creating firmer, smoother skin, which diminishes the appearance of scars and produces an overall clearer complexion. The injectable gel is made up of 80 percent purified collagen. In clinical studies Bellafill's efficacy was observed for as long as twelve months. The most common local side effects are swelling, bruising, redness, pain, discoloration, itching, and hardness of the skin. Some patients experienced headaches, swelling of the side of the nose, moderate cold sores, lip numbness, and lip dryness. These side effects were often mild to moderate and most resolved within one week.

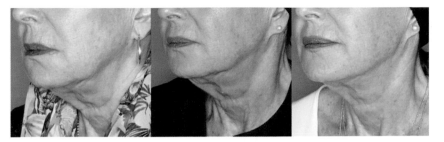

Before and after of nonsurgical neck lift using Kybella, fillers, lasers, and neuromodulators.

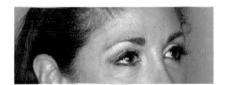 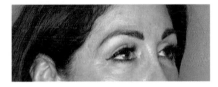

Before and after of nonsurgical brow lift using Ultherapy, fillers, and neuromodulators.

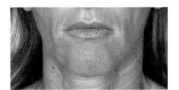 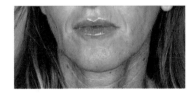

Before and after of perioral rejuvenation using hyaluronic acid fillers and neuromodulators.

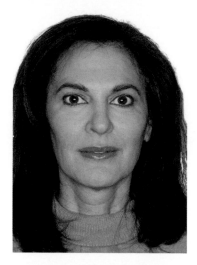

The facial expressions we make engage various facial muscles repeatedly over a lifetime and eventually cause lines.

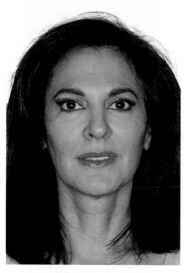

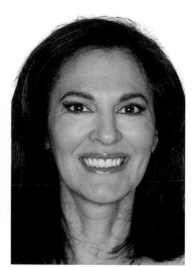

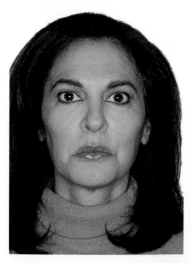

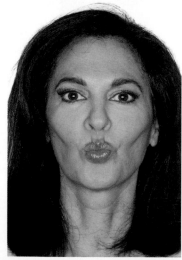

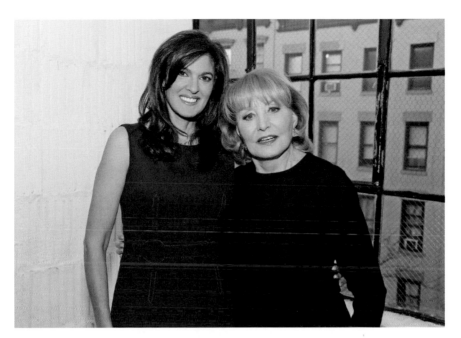

With Barbara Walters after filming the 20/20 special "The Cutting Edge."
(© *American Broadcasting Companies, Inc.*)

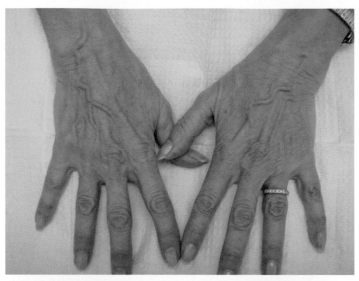

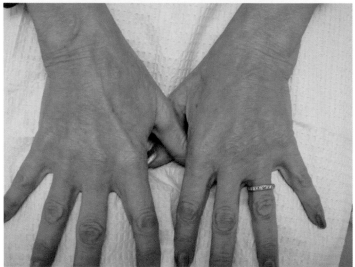

Before and after of hands treated with Radiesse injections to dramatically soften the appearance of prominent veins and tendons, for younger-looking hands.

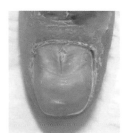

A cracked nail as a result of repetitive trauma called "habit tic deformity."

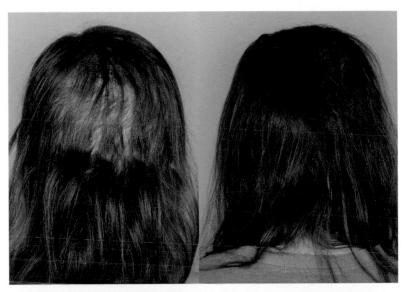

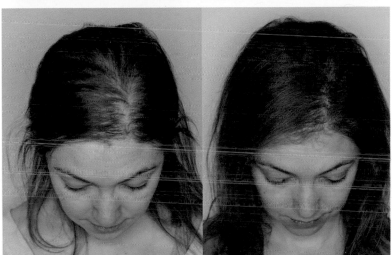

The dramatic hair regrowth, after persistent treatment including PRP (platelet-rich plasma) injections, was life-changing for this patient.

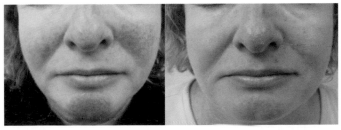

A patient with rosacea before and after IPL (intense pulsed light) treatment.

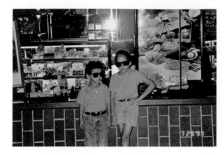

A fond memory of my son, Andrew, and daughter, Sabrina, in childhood. They have my heart, give me so much joy, and help me remember to savor the moment.

The antidote to a stressful day: spending time with "Baby," my therapy dog who has also lifted the spirits of my patients on many occasions.

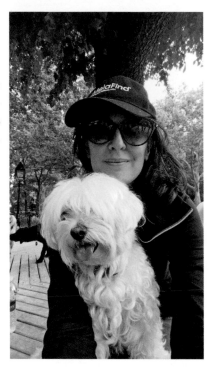

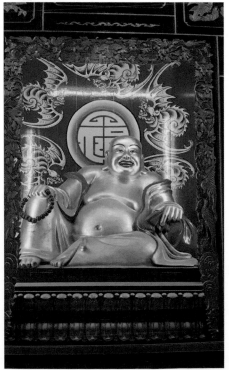

Laughter is good for your soul, your body, and your skin! Benefits of laughter have been recognized across the ages and cultures. Here's a photo of a laughing Buddha, my favorite Buddha, from a recent trip to Thailand.

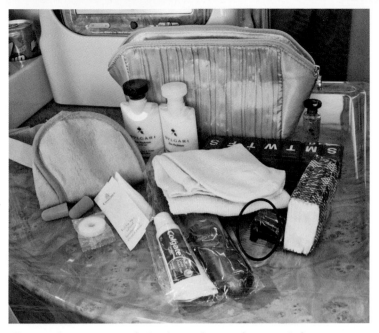

The on-the-go essentials I take with me whenever I fly.

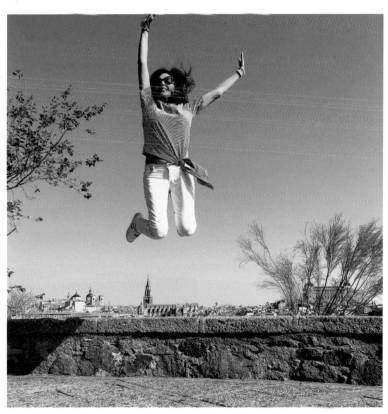

I love exploring new places and studying ingredients for products! Here is my mountain jump on a recent investigative trip to Spain.

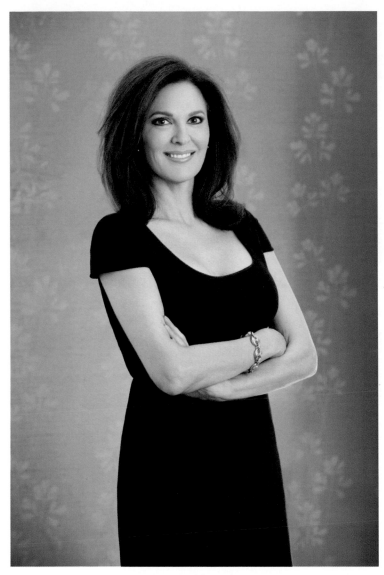

I hope you use my prescription for feeling Beyond Beautiful and that you make every day the #bestDAYever. *(credit: Jonathan R. Beckerman)*

Hyaluronic acid fillers can help to temporarily improve acne scars and may have permanent results over time, since the injection is often combined with subcision, which breaks up the bound-down damaged collagen and helps to replace it with healthy younger collagen.

Sculptra is made of poly-L-lactic acid, an ingredient found in absorbable stiches. This is one of my favorite products. I have found treatment with Sculptra to be a great starting point for my patients with multiple deep acne scars. Results normally last two to four years, but I have found them to be even longer-lasting in most patients.

Lasers and Devices

There are outstanding treatments available, from the classical CO2 laser that blasts away scars to the newer Pico or sound wave devices, along with fractional lasers and microneedling, with or without radio-frequency energy, for any type of acne scar. The end result will be smoother but not perfect skin. Treatments usually need to be done in a series, but the results can be dramatic and quite beautiful.

ASK DR. DAY

Q: *I've had acne since I was thirteen and I'm now forty-six. I eat a vegan diet, and I'm conscious of my stress levels and how much sleep I get. I've taken Accutane five times over the years, but my acne seems to be getting worse, and I feel like it's hormonally related. I've even done Fraxel laser treatments, and I'm using an antibiotic/retinol combo. My doctor wants to put me back on the Accutane. It works for about a year, then the acne comes back with a vengeance. What do you think I should do?*

DD: It's just not fair to have to battle wrinkles and pimples at the same time! Actually, chances are you don't have a lot of wrinkles because your skin is oily, so that's a good thing. I suggest asking your dermatologist about spironolactone. It's FDA-approved as a diuretic, but it also blocks certain hormone receptors, which is how it helps with acne. It's one of my favorite and most reliable treatments for adult acne (even if it's off-label), because it's not a hormone or an antibiotic and has little in the way of side effects at the dosages used for acne. It takes about three months to see a significant difference. Tazorac is a gel that also seems to work well. Low dose oral isotretinoin (better known under the brand name Accutane) can also be helpful. A 10 mg pill twice a week may be an off-label but effective way to keep the oil production in check.

Salicylic acid in the form of a lotion or in your face wash is also excellent to help control oil and minimize the appearance of pores. Be sure to wear a light hydrator rather than moisturizer and look for sunscreen in the form of a gel or powder to avoid clogging pores. A hydrator will help with water balance without being occlusive. A great example of a hydrator is hyaluronic acid. It helps hold and pull water into your skin. Try the SkinCeuticals H.A. Intensifier to help hydrate your skin as you treat the acne.

WHAT IS ROSACEA?

Rosacea is a condition that often takes people by surprise. Because it doesn't start in childhood, most people don't even think of it. It often first starts during a person's thirties or later and seems to worsen at the most inconvenient times, like when you're stressed because you're about to give a big presentation, or when you're out celebrating and having a few drinks with friends, or on a date. One of the most common things patients say when I diagnose rosacea is "How can I have rosacea? I never had it as a child." My answer is: "The good news is you didn't have it sooner!" Some skin conditions, like rosacea, don't appear until you reach adulthood. A family history of rosacea could be a clue that you're prone to it. Also, on the good news side is that it's not necessarily a progressive condition; and while we can't cure it, there are excellent treatments available to help control it.

Many people mistake rosacea as acne and treat it with antiacne medications, many of which only make the problem worse. While acne has a bacteria as a main root cause, rosacea is more inflammatory in nature. If you are one of those people who blush easily and turn "beet red" when you are embarrassed, or you break out after drinking alcohol or eating certain foods, then you may be one of the millions who have rosacea. Rosacea can occur in any ethnicity, and most forms are more common in women than in men.

It's important to have an evaluation of redness of the face because there are several possible conditions that can cause this, some of which may be serious, and early diagnosis and treatment can make a big difference in outcome.

Here are the four different types of rosacea, along with treatment options:

1. Papules and Pustules

Known as the acne rosacea or the rosacea breakout, these are red bumps and pustules that appear, usually in the center of the face, the forehead, and around the mouth. It can look like acne, but without blackheads and whiteheads.

Treatment includes over-the-counter products that contain sulfa, azelaic acid, or prescription-strength versions of the same. These medications may be used alone or in combination with other prescriptions, such as oral antibiotics that are used more for their anti-inflammatory than antibiotic effect, and topicals such as metronidazole or ivermectin.

Chemical Peels. There are also chemical peels specifically designed for treating rosacea skin. They can help with breakouts, restore the water balance, and repair the skin barrier that is often damaged in skin with rosacea.

2. Redness, Flushing, and Broken Blood Vessels

Rosacea with these types of symptoms can be treated with lasers, like the pulsed dye laser, and devices such as intense pulsed light (IPL) or broadband light that target the redness. Though there is little to no downtime, a series of treatments is required and often needs to be repeated over time to maintain the results.

Mirvaso and Rhofade. These topical prescription treatments are FDA-approved to temporarily reduce the redness of rosacea. Applied to the face in the morning, calming effects begin after about thirty minutes and wear off at about twelve hours. Mirvaso was the first to become available and I have many patients who swear by it, but in a minority of patients there may be a rebound redness, which leaves the skin redder as the effect of the medication wears off. Rhofade is a newer formulation in the anti-redness category and has provided excellent results in reducing redness with little to no rebound effect.

3. Rhinophyma

Think W. C. Fields's nose. This is the one type of rosacea more common in men and more associated with drinking alcohol. The nose looks full, red, and bulbous. It can be treated with lasers, radio-frequency energy, and surgery, but avoiding triggers is also very helpful.

4. Ocular Rosacea

Up to 50 percent of those suffering from rosacea may also have eye involvement, seen as styes, a gritty feeling in the eyes known as blepharitis, redness of the eyes, and light sensitivity. Ocular rosacea can lead to blindness if not treated. It is important to see an ophthalmologist as soon as possible if you have symptoms of ocular rosacea.

In-office treatments for all but the occular forms of rosacea include:

- **Pulsed Dye Laser.** The Vbeam is one of the most popular lasers used in our practice. It is an advanced pulsed dye laser that targets redness and is helpful in treating both roseacea and sun damage on the face, neck, and chest. The light is absorbed by the blood vessels in the skin; these blood vessels are then reabsorbed by the body, allowing for a cleaner, more refreshed appearance with fewer visible pores.

- **Red Light Therapy.** NASA scientists and dermatologists have discovered red light therapy to promote faster cell growth using infrared light wavelengths. Safe, visible, infrared light wavelengths penetrate the skin and stimulate the production of natural enzymes that in turn increase collagen production and reduce inflammation. Red light therapy smooths overall skin tone, repairs sun damage, and helps reduce redness, flushing, and broken capillaries. In addition to building collagen, this therapy also helps to fade stretch marks and scars, and aids in reducing fine lines, wrinkles, crow's-feet, laugh lines, and under-eye wrinkles.

As with every condition I report to you, I want to make sure you pay attention to how connected your mind, body, and skin are, and this is especially important if you have rosacea. My lovely patient Helen is the perfect example.

Helen is a long-standing cosmetic patient. She has beautiful skin of color, takes great care of her skin, comes in regularly for fillers and neuromodulators, and is aging beautifully. On one recent visit I walked into the examination room and was surprised to see her face flushed red and broken out. Something was definitely up. I asked how she was doing and how I could help. She told me her face kept getting redder and had started to break out. She said she had tried a number of over-the-counter treatments for acne, but everything she did only made it worse.

I explained that she had rosacea and this was different from acne and needed different treatments. When I asked how long it had been going on, she replied, "Six weeks," which was a pretty precise answer. Most people say vaguer things like, "Awhile," or, "On and off," but very few will give me such a specific number of weeks or have the answer so readily available. She knew exactly when it started and she knew why. Now it was my turn to help her solve the issue for the best results. I reviewed rosacea with her, as I have described here for you, and we discussed appropriate treatments. But it was important to see if there was more to the story, so I asked her what might have happened six weeks ago to trigger the breakout. She looked at me and said, "I knew you'd go there." She told me that six weeks ago her youngest sister had died of lung cancer. Helen was the oldest of three sisters and they were all very close. She had taken the loss very hard, and of course it made sense that her rosacea had flared. But that didn't fully explain it; I knew there had to be more to the story, so I pressed on.

We talked about what had happened and how present she was from the time of her sister's diagnosis until the end. She explained that she was happy she had been able to be there, but it was difficult because her sister had lived in a town two hours away and received treatment in a hospital there. Helen was lucky because her husband was very supportive and had often even accompanied her on her visits. However, it had been stressful juggling work and family and so difficult to watch her sister suffer.

Then, Helen told me something surprising. Although she spoke very casually, I watched her face turn redder and redder as she spoke. She told me that several months before her sister was diagnosed, the three sisters had gone on vacation together. While on holiday the two older sisters had noticed that their younger sister had lost some weight and mentioned she should go in for a checkup. But their sister had insisted everything was fine and that she felt great.

I pointed out that she seemed to be angry at her sister for not listening to her advice to get a checkup. She looked at me, stunned, and said, "You're right! I am mad!" She hadn't let herself dwell on that memory because it was too painful and agonizing to think that if only she had continued to push her sister to get checked out, or if only her sister had listened, the cancer could have been diagnosed sooner, and her sister might still be here today. Helen's appearance conveyed an important and powerful message: Her grief was clearly complicated, and without fully addressing it, all the other treatments would only cover up the issue rather than help to resolve it in a more lasting way. She would miss the opportunity to truly heal in the way her body was trying to guide her. We spoke about the best treatments, but also about the opportunity to pay attention to what her body was telling her and to explore ways to deal with it so she could truly heal and also honor the memory of her sister in the best way possible.

ROSACEA TRIGGERS

The exact cause of rosacea remains a mystery. However, one theory is the mite theory, which posits that bacteria associated with increased numbers of demodex mites in the pores of the face may aggravate the skin by affecting the pH and the local skin microbiome, which can cause redness and inflammation.

We may not know the exact cause of rosacea, but we do know there are triggers; and one way to keep rosacea at bay is to avoid or better manage them. I confess that I have rosacea and my personal trigger is vinegar. You know when you have a personal trigger, because within hours to a day after consuming or having contact with that trigger, you see the rash come through.

Alcoholic beverages, hot drinks, hot and spicy foods, dairy products. Alcohol is one of the biggest triggers, and new studies have shown that white wine may be more of a trigger than red, but you'll know if and when you have had too much because you'll see a flare-up of your rosacea. As I mentioned, alcohol also increases the risk of rhinophyma, which is a form of rosacea causing fullness and distortion of the nose.

Spicy foods and dairy have also been known to trigger rosacea, but these are more commonly personal triggers. It might help to keep a diary of your flares to see if you can discern a pattern.

Stress and anxiety. Take note (in your Face Book, perhaps) of your emotional state before and during rosacea breakouts. Were you particularly anxious on that day? Did you just have a fight with your spouse or partner? Was work especially challenging? Stress is definitely a trigger for this condition, so read my chapter on "Mindful Beauty" and follow some of the Beyond Beautiful relaxation techniques during periods of emotional turbulence.

Extremes in temperature. Sun, strong wind, and going from hot or cold outdoors to the opposite indoors all can trigger rosacea.

10 COMMON CAUSES OF SKIN RASHES

Rashes can be both maddening and embarrassing. They are caused by a seemingly infinite number of factors, including environment, infection, stress, heat, allergens, immune system disorders, and medication. Many clear up on their own; however, more chronic skin conditions, such as dermatitis and eczema, might require a visit to your doctor for medication or treatment.

Here are the ten most common annoying culprits responsible for skin rashes:

1. Perfumed Soap and Products

Your skin has its own special microbiome. This is the environment of microbes that help your skin look its best. Harsh soaps and detergents can strip the skin and leave it sensitive and irritated. If you are prone to eczema, it can have a worsening effect. The solution is simple: Use dye-free, perfume-free products. Look for fragrance-free, not unscented, as unscented may have a masking fragrance. Dye-free detergents such as All Free Clear laundry detergent, the Tide Free & Gentle line, and Seventh Generation detergent are excellent options. Seventh Generation is an Environmental Protection Agency (EPA) Safer Choice certified product, made of 96 percent plant-based ingredients.

2. Genetics

As much as we love our families, and we can inherit many of their good qualities, our parents or grandparents can also pass down the propensity for rashes like eczema and allergies. If a parent suffers from psoriasis, for instance, chances are increased that a child may develop it as well.

3. Allergies

Seasonal allergies can also trigger a variety of skin reactions, like hives, that form itchy red bumps on the surface of the skin due to histamine release into the bloodstream. In some cases infections, foods, medications, alcohol, and additives can also cause hives. For children, the most frequent food allergy is to peanuts, thus all the nut-free schools. Some foods or exposures to chemicals can cause eczema, especially in children. Treatment often requires a multidisciplinary approach with your dermatologist, allergist, and pediatrician or internist.

4. Stress

I'm sure you are aware by now that some skin irritations, also known as dermatitis, are a direct result of anxiety. When we are stressed out the chemical process in the body turns up the heat, and this chemical reaction can trigger many skin conditions. Where and how skin irritation shows up will give you important clues as to what you need to pay attention to and change in order to be happier and more fulfilled. Every setback is a setup for success and growth. The reason I wrote this book was to parse the word *stress* beyond the generic, to help identify how specific stressors trigger what you see on your skin and how you feel about yourself.

5. Chemical Cleaners

Many household cleaners contain harsh chemicals, which are added to cut through grease and remove stains. I suggest wearing gloves if you use these products, even if it's only for a short amount of time. Consider switching to more environmentally friendly cleaning products, such as Honest Company brands, which are made with biodegradable, nontoxic ingredients and are cruelty-free (not tested on animals).

6. Plants

One of a camper's or hiker's worst nightmares (other than running into a hungry bear) is a brush with a patch of poison ivy, poison oak, or poison sumac. These plants can produce some of the most uncomfortable itchy, blistery rashes within a few days of exposure that last up to several weeks. The rashes are caused by an oil found in the plants. You have about ten minutes to wash it off after contact before it penetrates and makes the rash inevitable. The reaction is a toxic rather than an allergic reaction. Some people are more sensitive than others and will react sooner and more vigorously. I'm one of those and I can tell you from firsthand knowledge that it's very, very uncomfortable! Contrary to popular belief, the rash itself is not contagious and does not spread. What appears as spreading is actually a delayed reaction. If your face or eye begins to swell up, see a doctor right away. Your dermatologist will be able to give you prescription-strength medications.

7. Bites

The skin reactions to insect bites vary depending on the offender and your immunity. Stinging insects like bees will cause painful marks at the site of attack; whereas biters, like ants and spiders, will secrete venom that can irritate and even ulcerate the skin. Most bites and stings will heal on their own, but if you are allergic to bees and have an anaphylactic reaction, you must keep an EpiPen with you at all times and do anything you can to avoid exposure. Different tick bites can cause a variety of infections such as Lyme disease, borreliosis, erlichiosis, Powassan virus, and Rocky Mountain spotted fever. These infections sometimes show up with skin reactions at the site of the bite, including a generalized rash or the more distinctive bull's-eye rash of Lyme disease, so it's important to keep an eye out for any unusual marks or changes in your skin and seek the care of your dermatologist right away to avoid long-term issues.

There are various things you can do to relieve pain, itching, and swelling from mosquito or other bug bites: Apply a cold pack to the area. An antihistamine taken every six to twelve hours, depending on the brand, will give you some relief from the itching. Hydrocortisone 1 percent cream can also provide some relief. Your dermatologist can prescribe a stronger cortisone to help reduce inflammation faster. Topical lidocaine will help numb the spot temporarily. Scratching is the worst thing to do; it will only make the bite itch more and increases the risk of inflammation.

8. Heat Rash

A heat rash often develops in hot, overly sunny, or muggy weather, and is characterized by blisters or red lumps on the skin. The rash is the result of excessive sweating and friction (usually from skin or clothing) when sweat ducts are blocked and perspiration gets trapped under the skin. The rash will typically clear up in a few hours after you cool down. Try a cool shower or bath and let your skin air-dry. Don't use any type of oil-based product, which might block your sweat glands. Using a lotion with cortisone and taking antihistamines may also help calm the skin and relieve the discomfort.

9. Fabrics

Just about any material can cause irritation, especially for someone with sensitive skin—from your bath towel to your favorite sweater, especially if the fabric is abrasive, made with dark dyes (especially blue dye), chemical additives, or if it's too tight and is chafing against your skin. The most important things to look for when choosing fabrics that are good for sensitive skin are softness and breathability. Many synthetic fibers are prone to causing overheating or overcooling because they don't allow the skin to breathe. This can create conditions for bacterial and yeast growth that results in rashes and conditions like butt and back acne or an inflammation of the follicles called folliculitis. I see this every day in women who wear spandex, without underwear underneath, when they work out.

10. Cosmetics

Almost any beauty product you use has the potential to irritate your skin. There's really no such thing as hypoallergenic beauty products. All products are tested and designed to be as minimally allergenic as possible. The most common issues for allergies are preservatives and fragrance. One simple way to discern between an allergic (immune) reaction versus an irritant reaction is to put a dab of the offending product on the inside of your forearm. If you react, you are more likely to be allergic, and it may be worth seeing an allergist to determine the exact ingredients you are reacting to so you can avoid them in other products.

The Itchy and Scratchy Show (Eczema, Hives, Seborrhea)

Some of the most common chronic skin conditions that I treat in my office are not life-threatening but can create extreme discomfort and embarrassment. Some are inherited, some are caused by environmental and food allergies, and just about all of them are exacerbated by stress or some unresolved issues in our lives.

ECZEMA

This chronic immune related skin condition also tends to run in families. I think of it as an itch that rashes, meaning the itch comes up first and is exquisitely unbearable, making scratching unavoidable. The scratching leads to the rash. There are new treatments available called biologics for moderate to severe eczema in adults, and the relief is very welcome to those who suffer from this condition. Keeping the skin healthy and intact is very important, which means avoiding long, hot showers and moisturizing at least twice a day. Antihistamines and topical cortisone also help to control the itch and can break the itch-scratch cycles.

HIVES

Hives are red, itchy, raised areas of skin that appear in varying shapes and sizes and typically last less than twenty-four hours in any given spot.

They are caused by an immune reaction in which white blood cells called mast cells release histamine into the blood in response to a perceived, but misguided, need to protect the body. Since this reaction can be brought on by such a large variety of exposures and usually resolves without treatment within six weeks, we don't usually even start to investigate the possible cause until after six weeks, when hives are considered chronic. Causes can range from a viral infection, to parasites, to a reaction to a medication, food, heat, cold, or even touch, so the investigation can take time and require coordination with an allergist. There's also a type of hives called dermatographism. In this case, anytime you scratch or even touch the skin, you develop a hive in that spot. The underlying cause is unknown, and the hives can last for weeks to years.

Treatments include antihistamines to give sufferers some relief until the hives go away. It can take a few days for these to work, and you have to take them regularly in order to inhibit the release of histamines into the blood by the mast cells. In serious or extensive cases, a course of an oral steroid called prednisone may be needed to help suppress the hives until the body gets past the trigger.

SEBORRHEIC DERMATITIS

If you have a red, itchy, scaly rash on your scalp, it could be seborrhea, also known as seborrheic dermatitis. This common skin disease appears similar to psoriasis, eczema, or an allergic reaction. It can appear on other parts of the body as well, such as the brows, the sides of the nose, and the chest. Sometimes, seborrhea will clear up by itself. More often, though, treatment is required to control it, as well as focusing on how your skin considers the triggers that may cause flares. Treatments include topical steroids; shampoos that contain salicylic acid or zinc pyrithione; or antifungal shampoos such as Nizoral.

ASK DR. DAY

Q: *I've been getting rashes under my arms, which I think are from shaving more often. Are there types of deodorants or ingredients I should or shouldn't be using?*

DD: Rashes in the armpit are usually signs of irritation from shaving, deodorants/antiperspirants, and/or sweat. If the rash spares the armpit but affects the skin directly around the armpit, it is most likely due to clothing or something rubbing against the skin. Here's the scoop: The skin under the arms is more sensitive than the surrounding skin. It is also an area that is naturally occluded by the arm hanging down over it, so anything applied to the skin sinks in more quickly and can be more irritating. It is also an area that is typically moist from sweat and products that break down sweat, which can be irritating to the skin. So, if there are any breaks in the skin from scratching or shaving, yeast and bacteria can overgrow and make the itching/redness worse. Antiperspirants are by necessity acidic to help them penetrate the sweat glands and to be effective in stopping sweating. If you apply an antiperspirant to freshly shaved skin, not only can it sting and burn, but it can also make the skin turn red and become inflamed. Shaving dry skin or shaving wet skin without proper shaving cream or lubrication, can cause micro-breaks in the skin. When you sweat, the urea and ammonia from the perspiration can irritate the skin. The problem is compounded by the fact that most people use the same shaver for too long, after it has at least a few dull spots, which may also cause micro-nicks to the skin.

Try changing your routine so that you shave at night, change razors more frequently, and be sure to wash off any remaining antiperspirant at the end of each day.

If you do get a rash, try using 1 percent hydrocortisone with aloe to soothe the skin. If it does not improve within one week, see your dermatologist for a prescription-strength cortisone or possibly an anti-yeast medication. Look for antiperspirants that are fragrance-free, not unscented. Fragrance-free means there is no fragrance. Unscented means the product has no smell, but it may contain a masking fragrance. If you run out of shaving cream or gel, try using conditioner as a substitute. It's better and softer than soap or shampoo.

Coming up...check out the next chapter on "Mindful Beauty." We all know that the mind and the body are inextricably connected. There are scientifically proven methods for reducing our anxiety, which in turn improves our health, our skin, and our well-being.

CHAPTER NINE

Mindful Beauty

*Ten Steps to Reduce Stress, Feel Better, and Look
More Beautiful*

"The best and most beautiful things in the world cannot be
seen or even touched—they must be felt with the heart."
—*Helen Keller*

Your relationship with yourself affects and controls the world around
you. "Mindful beauty" and my concept of Beyond Beautiful are about
having control over the way you see yourself and how others see you.
Being happy is a choice, feeling and seeing beauty in yourself and in
the world around you is also a choice and, in this chapter, I will help
you understand how obvious and easy a choice it is to make.

Did you know the part of our brain that recognizes faces increases
in weight as we age, unlike other parts of the brain, such as those that
discern places? This helps us perceive differences between friend and
foe, but it also helps us to recognize nuances that influence how we
see ourselves and how we see beauty. Much of the treatment involved
when I help restore and rejuvenate my patients involves creating a
balance of light and shadow and is not obvious on the surface but
looks natural and beautiful, because these subtleties are definitively
recognized by the brain.

When I was a kid learning to ride a bicycle, my mom could see I was having a hard time. I kept looking at the ground to make sure I wasn't going to fall. She told me, "Look where you want to go. If you look down, you'll fall; if you look left, you'll go left." Her words were like magic. I looked forward and aimed for my uncle, who was waiting for me at the end of the block, and off I went. My balance came naturally. My body did what it needed to do to keep me on the bike, and my feet pedaled fast enough to keep me moving forward.

The advice she gave helped me learn to ride a bike, but I have thought about her words and their greater meaning over the years, as well as the advice of one of my dad's patients who was a teacher.

I liked to think of myself as my dad's youngest medical apprentice. I used to wake up at 5 a.m., have him sing "Que Sera, Sera" to me as he shaved, and have breakfast with him before he walked across the street to NYU hospital to take care of his patients. Even as a young girl, he would occasionally take me with him on rounds. I usually sat at the nurses' station, but sometimes he let me see patients with him if he thought we would both benefit from the experience.

One of the patients I met was a teacher. He knew she didn't have family of her own or anyone to visit. He also knew she was a wise woman and had great advice, so he brought me in to see her, too, as he went in to discharge her home. We sat and chatted for a while, she asked some questions about me, and I enjoyed hearing her talk about her experience with my dad. I was proud to know he was so loved by his patients, and so caring and gentle. As I got up to leave, she said, "I want you to always remember to keep your chin up; you will get there, and anywhere you want to go." Her advice was similar to my mom's; essentially, that if you focus on your goal and see yourself where you need to be, you will get there.

Fast-forward many years to medical school, when I took an elective on hypnosis. On the first day of class the professor hypnotized me, and in my hypnotic trance he had me act and feel as if I were drunk. He asked me a series of questions while I was under. I could hear myself answering his questions with slurred speech; I could feel myself following his commands voluntarily and believing I chose and wanted to do the things he suggested, like walking across the room backward and other benign but odd tasks, wobbling as if completely bombed, even though I had not had a drop of alcohol. He brought me out of the hypnotized state, leaving me with full awareness of the experience, and also taught me how to hypnotize myself. At the time I was amazed at the experience. I recalled all of it and found it remarkable that it was possible. I began to realize how much of life was in my head, how much "believing is seeing" rather than "seeing is believing." Each of our experiences emphasizes the value and power of our vision of, and relationship with, ourselves.

This is also true of how we see ourselves when we look in the mirror or in the mirror of our mind's eye. If you are searching for a magic lotion or potion that will make your skin look healthier and more vibrant, I can honestly tell you that the answer lies, in part, inside your head. The mind is the key to improving every facet of your life and has the immense power to make you look and feel your best. Your brain generates thoughts, emotions, actions, reactions, moods, dreams, and creative ideas. It holds all the memories, experiences, and knowledge that you have accumulated since you drew your first breath. It interprets every sensation you experience and controls each movement you make. What you think and what you feel is all based on the fact that the mind is part of the body, and they function as one unit. When you're anxious you get pale, and when you're angry or embarrassed your face gets red. Your mind is your essence, and it is also the essence of mindful beauty. The care and "feeding" of your mind will make you feel more energized and alive—all of which makes you more beautiful!

The following is my eleven-step program for achieving mindful beauty. If you can't follow all the steps initially, then tackle them one by one. I guarantee that each step will help alleviate some of the anxiety that comes with everyday living and, ultimately, allow you to see a transformation in the overall health of your skin and body.

STEP ONE: UNPLUG

Our social networks help us stay connected to friends and family, but they can also alienate and isolate us. It's becoming a bigger problem as we expand from texts and e-mail to Facebook, Instagram, Twitter, Snapchat, YouTube, and more—there's not enough time in the day to keep up! We've all seen this situation, or maybe even been part of it ourselves: sitting in a room or around a dinner table with people who are too busy staring at their devices to engage in conversation. It not only creates sensations of depression and anxiety, it also creates tech neck and bad facial posture, both of which age us beyond our years. I see people squinting and frowning at the screen as they sit hunched over, staring at it for hours at a time. We now know that many of the apps are designed to be addictive, because getting more likes or responses makes you happy, at least for the moment, and keeps you coming back for more. It's an endless cycle that takes you away from being active in your environment. And it can affect your breathing, which affects your health, since shallower and shorter breaths give less oxygen and can make you feel tired and anxious.

While not everyone develops an Internet and smartphone addiction, having a strong dependence on your devices is definitely a warning sign that you need to at least curb your enthusiasm for online activities.

Here are some ways to break the Internet habit:

Set limits. Psychologists recommend that you spend no more than an hour or two a day using the Internet for anything other than work or school.

Create a schedule. Set certain times during the day to check your e-mail when you're not working and do not exceed that self-imposed limit. Checking once every two hours seems reasonable.

Turn off your alerts. If your smartphone pings every time someone e-mails, texts, or posts, you'll be continually checking your phone. Change your settings to prevent immediate notifications.

Use some selfie-control. Take time to be in the moment when sightseeing or going to a concert before you take photos, selfies, send an Instagram, Snapchat, tweet, or go live on Facebook.

Check your emotions instead of your e-mail. When you're using the Internet, take a moment to write down how you are feeling. Similarly, when you're not using it, but are craving a game of *Candy Crush*, write down how you are feeling. An "addiction journal" will give you some insight into how your Internet craving is affecting your emotional health.

Institute a no-phone zone at the dinner table at home or at a restaurant. If you must text, e-mail, or call when you are sitting down to eat, excuse yourself and find a private place to use your phone.

Stop being rude. Never look at your screen while you are engaged in a conversation with someone (that's like saying there's someone or something more important than the person you're with).

Stop engaging in risky behavior. For your own safety (and that of others), do not look at your device while walking up and down the stairs or crossing the street, and never, ever text while driving! No exceptions. Pull over.

Make amends. If your children, friends, or family have busted you about your phone addiction, apologize and promise to change your behavior. Make good on your word by taking the person you offended out for lunch or dinner, and shut off your phone.

Reward good behavior. Give yourself a reward at the end of the week for sticking to the program by putting $20 (or whatever amount you choose) in a jar or savings account. Buy yourself something nice at the end of the month with the money you've saved.

Get help. If you have a serious addiction, find a support group. Depending on where you live, you may be able to attend a meeting of Internet and Technology Addiction Anonymous (ITAA).

STEP TWO: GET A SOCIAL LIFE

I have built a family of "Derm Diva Sisters" whom I frequently see at dermatological events around the country and around the world. They are an incredible group of brilliant, beautiful, and accomplished women. They have become family, and the best part is we have much in common through our passion for our work and our goals for balanced life fulfillment: to be at the top of our specialty, and to have time for our families and friends. We all support and celebrate one another through good times, rally to help one another through bad times, and, as a group we embody a wide range of personality types and opinions—so there's never a dull moment!

I encourage you to introduce more friends, acquaintances, family, and fun into your life. Having an active social life has been proven to improve overall health as well as the health of your skin. Many studies have shown that it might also increase your longevity! The more social we are throughout our lives, the less likely we are to suffer mental and physical decline as we age, all of which helps us to maintain a more youthful appearance.

Here are some ideas:

Make a new friend. Believe it or not, making new friendships is a great way to keep you feeling younger and looking better. Unlike children, who are continually meeting and making new friends, adults tend to get stuck in a social rut and to run with the same crowd they've been with for years. While longtime friendships should be cherished, it is good for our health and vitality to at least occasionally seek out one new friend, or possibly reconnect with someone you haven't seen in a while. If you don't know where to start, go to meetup.com, which has group gatherings in your local community based on shared interests (much like my Derm Divas). It runs the gamut in terms of age and passions, from millennials to boomers, book readers to board gamers, microbrewers to wine tasters, and tennis players to chess masters. Pick a group and start bonding! Socializing with friends can change the way we feel about ourselves and the way we interact with the world at large.

Mix it up. Widen your social circle by allowing yourself to befriend people who have opinions and ideas different from your own. Taking ourselves out of our comfort zone makes life more exciting.

Beware of toxic friends. Think about the relationships in your life that zap you of your confidence and prevent you from reaching your full potential, physically and emotionally. They may not be bad people; they're just bad for you. The more time you spend with people like this, the worse you will feel about yourself. This kind of negativity is contagious and will show on your face and in your posture. If you're in a relationship with a toxic person, the sooner you allow yourself to recognize it and separate yourself from it, the better.

Keep close ties with friends and family. In his book *Outliers*, Malcolm Gladwell writes about the groundbreaking study of a group of Italian immigrants who lived in Roseto, Pennsylvania, named for the village south of Rome where they came from: "In Roseto, virtually no one under fifty-five died of a heart attack, or showed any signs of heart disease," Gladwell writes. For men over sixty-five, the death rate from heart disease in Roseto was roughly half that of the United States as a whole.

Stewart Wolf, MD, who taught at the University of Oklahoma, enlisted students, colleagues, and sociologists to help with his investigation of why people from this town fared so well. After a detailed and very in-depth investigation, the results were surprisingly simple. Wolf concluded that the answer lay in the way the Rosetans lived. Men and women stopped to chat on the street; they cooked for one another and gathered in their backyards. Many homes had three family generations living under one roof. They went to church regularly and there were no less than twenty-two civic organizations among them. The towns-people also discouraged the wealthier residents (not that there were many) from flaunting their success and encouraged them to help the less fortunate.

In short, Rosetans were healthy because they were a close-knit and social people. The transplanted *paesani* culture of southern Italy created a nurturing, protective, social cocoon of sorts, where caring for one's neighbor inoculated residents from debilitating stress and the pressures of the modern world.

STEP THREE: GET MOVING!

You already know that exercise is good for your heart and lungs, but did you know that it's also good for your skin and your face? A Finnish study of middle-aged athletes showed that the participants who exercised had noticeably fewer wrinkles than the sedentary control group. The active athletes' skin was not as thin as the skin of those in the sedentary group, and it tended to be far more resilient. The Scandinavian scientists concluded that the reason for the positive effects of exercise on aging skin is that cells in the layer where new skin is formed speed up their activity. In other words, when you get moving, so do your cells! Countless studies have also shown that people who boost their heart rates through exercise, especially interval training, lower their risk of depression and stress. Why does exercise keep us so calm? The increased blood flow that comes with physical activity releases feel-good neurotransmitters, including endorphins, the brain's natural chemicals that produce feelings of happiness and well-being. The good news for all you exercise-haters out there is that you don't have to run a marathon or join a gym to reap the mental benefits. Research has found that as little as twenty minutes of physical activity, including a brisk walk, can do the trick (although longer is better). The art of play also counts and has the added benefit of improving creativity and thought as well as friendships. Find a sport you like and get involved!

Here's another reason that moving is key to maintaining healthy skin: Anything that promotes circulation also helps your skin to look more vibrant. In addition to providing oxygen and blood flow, which helps to nourish skin cells, exercise also helps carry away any waste products, including free radicals, from working cells. Think of it as cleansing your skin from the inside. Even conditions that are exacerbated by stress, such as hives, rashes, and eczema, can show some improvement after working out. The facial yoga exercises I've described in this book should be done along with body yoga, Pilates, weight training, or any other exercise you choose. They may be your best and least expensive wrinkle fighter yet!

Exercise Caution

I can't think of a reason not to exercise throughout your lifetime, given that you are in good health and are physically able, but there are a few caveats. I highly recommend that you see a doctor before you start any new physical routine if you have health issues or if you haven't exercised in a long time or ever.

Any time you exercise or spend time outdoors, be sure to wear sunscreen (apply it liberally) with an SPF of at least 30. Sunburns and sun damage increase the potential of getting skin cancer and can rapidly age the skin, erasing any benefits your skin might obtain from your outdoor workouts. I suggest that you avoid exercising outside during the peak sun-exposure time of 10 a.m. to 4 p.m. There are newer sunscreens available that don't sting your eyes. If you have oily skin or problems with acne, choose a gel or oil-free product, a sports block gel, or the latest powder laced with SPF protection.

But don't count on sunscreen alone to protect you if you're spending hours in the sun or swimming. Sweating and water can remove the sunscreen that you put on, and there is evidence that sweating actually increases the chances of sunburn. If you are sweating, it can take as much as 40 percent less ultraviolet rays to burn than when you do not break a sweat. Wear sun-protective workout clothing that covers as much skin as possible and a broad-brimmed hat to shade your face.

Another skin problem that may develop during physical activity is chafing, which can cause rashes. For people prone to acne, the irritation and increased perspiration produced by tight-fitting workout clothes may lead to an acne attack. If you suffer from this kind of breakout, wear moisture-wicking clothing, including sports bras and hats, to keep skin drier and cooler, and shower immediately after exercising. Wearing loose-fitting workout clothes will also help. Be sure your skin is clean before you exercise to prevent clogged pores that lead to acne, and avoid wearing makeup. After showering, apply a soothing skin moisturizer or powder to help prevent skin irritation.

STEP FOUR: RELAX AND RESTORE

Relaxation protects our spirit in the same way that sunscreen protects our skin. Healthy forms of relaxation reduce stress, thus lowering the skin-damaging levels of cortisol (the stress hormone). Unfortunately, many people try to ease stress with unhealthy habits such as overeating, especially "comfort" foods, drinking too much alcohol, and smoking. While these attempts at coping with anxiety may temporarily calm us, in the long run they will create more misery, more remorse, and sallow, prematurely aging skin! I've included a section titled "Mindful Eating" in this chapter, along with an interview with registered dietitian Samantha Heller, author of *The Only Cleanse*.

The following actions have been scientifically proven to help us slow down, relax, elevate our mood, and reduce stress:

The Power of Touch. Massages can do more than make you relaxed and rejuvenated. Facial or cosmetic massages have been shown to improve the appearance of the skin for a short period of time after a treatment. This is due to an increase in blood flow and, ultimately, a spike in cellular oxygenation. As with many aspects of the skin, circulation decreases with age, leading to a dull complexion.

Meditate (Just Breathe). Modern medicine has embraced mindfulness and meditation as legitimate paths to relaxation and healing. These results, as you know by now, translate into ageless skin. In a world rife with quick fixes and magic pills, it's nice to know there is a scientifically proven practice that can truly change your life (or at least produce dramatic effects) in as little as ten to twenty-five minutes a day.

Yogis and researchers agree: meditating relaxes the brain, reduces anxiety, and decreases depression. Practitioners swear by its stress-relieving effects that can show up on our faces. This is supported by scores of studies, which continue to indicate that the ancient practice of meditation can help with pain and insomnia, and there's increasing evidence that it can even prevent some diseases by boosting the immune system.

Longtime meditators have also shown improved brain function resulting from a firing up of the neurons, and this increased activity in the prefrontal cortex is associated with positive emotions such as happiness. Meditation works by quieting the constant internal and external prattling in our heads. It can be as simple as sitting quietly and focusing on your breath or a mantra (a meaningful word or phrase). There are numerous traditions and no one way to meditate, so find a practice that works for you and do your best to stick with it.

I recommend reading *The Art of Happiness* by the Dalai Lama. You can also download the Headspace app, which has free guided meditations (https://www.headspace.com/). Oprah Winfrey and Deepak Chopra also offer free twenty-one-day guided meditations (https://chopracentermeditation.com/).

Take a Nature Walk. I agree with the American naturalist John Muir, who said, "In every walk with nature one receives more than he seeks." Think about how you feel when you hear such peaceful sounds of nature as birdsong, the rustling of leaves in the wind, the rolling waves of the ocean, the gentle babbling of a brook, or the rush of a waterfall. Whenever I am in nature I can feel my stress melting away like a snowflake in the sun.

Whenever possible, get away from the cacophony of ringtones, traffic, sirens, and other sights and sounds that assault your peace of mind. Take a nature walk in the woods, on a beach, or in your own backyard or garden. Research confirms a link between the amount of time we spend in nature, or in homes and workplaces with nature-based designs, and a reduction of stress and depression, a faster healing process, and less need for pain medication.

Get a pet. If you're an animal lover like me, you won't be surprised to learn that having a pet can also help lower your blood pressure and reduce your anxiety. There's something incredibly comforting about coming home after a long day at work and being greeted with the slobbery kisses of a dog or the loving rub of a furry purry cat. For many people, interacting with a pet is the ultimate antidote to a stressful day.

One thing I love about sharing my name with Doris Day is that we're both animal advocates. My little one is named Baby. He's a therapy dog, and in his younger years he would come to the office to see patients, by appointment, of course. I thought it would be mostly children who would be interested, but it turns out it was the adults who needed him the most. There were times Baby would go to the waiting room to greet patients, and when the patient came into the exam room, he or she would tell me how they were nervous about the visit or they were feeling down until Baby came directly to them. The touch and love the dog provided was needed and appreciated by my patients, and even to this day, years later, they still ask about him and hope he can come visit the office again soon. If you don't or can't have a pet of your own, see if you can volunteer at your local animal shelter; besides helping the animals, even brief encounters can create improvements in your mood. In one study, patients who spent a short amount of time with a dog before an operation experienced a 37 percent reduction in their anxiety levels, perhaps because the animal's presence helped distract them from their concerns.

Get Some Sleep. Unfortunately, there is no cream, pill, or procedure that can re-create what sleep does or compensate for the lack of it. Sound and restful sleep allows your skin to repair and rejuvenate. Most Americans are not getting enough sleep, which puts enormous stress on our bodies, our minds, and our skin. There has been some debate about the "right" amount of z's necessary for people to function properly during the day. Eight hours for adults used to be the magic number, but the National Sleep Foundation now says that not only do different age-groups need different amounts of sleep, but just like other characteristics we are born with, the amount of sleep we need to function well may differ from person to person. While you might be at your absolute best after sleeping seven hours a night, others might clearly need nine hours to live a happy, productive life. Sleeping long enough to go through four or five REM (rapid eye movement) cycles is probably the best measure for how long you should sleep. This is when you're dreaming the dreams you're most likely to remember.

Taking breaks is biologically restorative, but naps are even better (and are not just for babies and the elderly). In several studies, a nap of even ten minutes helped to improve brain function and decreased fatigue while reducing stressful cortisol levels. Parents know the importance of creating a sleep routine for kids, and the same goes for grown-ups. Going to bed and waking up at the same time is one way to create a good sleep ritual. To help you sleep, drink a hot cup of decaffeinated tea, listen to soothing music, burn some incense (lavender is said to have a calming effect), or do a little light reading before bedtime. Make sure your bedroom is as dark and quiet as possible, with no ambient light from phones, computers, or TVs. Sweet dreams!

STEP FIVE: CREATE

With all of life's responsibilities, we often forget that we need and deserve to take care of ourselves. Having a creative outlet, whatever it is and for however long you are able to do it, will make your self-esteem soar, and this spiritual rejuvenation will show on every pore of your body! A 2010 university study published in the *American Journal of Public Health* found that music, visual art therapy, dancing, and creative writing were effective in reducing some physiological and psychological disorders. This step requires you to stretch your creative muscles by dipping your toes or paintbrush into some of the activities mentioned below. Caveat: this means you must stop multitasking and immerse yourself in a single creative pursuit for between thirty and fifty minutes.

The Healing Power of Music. Music is the beat of my life. I find that there's a rhythm and a song for everything. Music can make me feel happy, or allow me to wallow in my misery when I need to. Think about the songs that bring tears to your eyes. Sometimes having a good cry can be a stress reliever. Every now and then a song from years ago will come on the radio and instantly take me back to my childhood and the beautiful memories of my sister. One of my favorites is "The Tears of a Clown." When I hear it I instantly go back in time and relive a happy lifetime moment with my sister. I feel Adriane's energy and realize she's always with me, and my love for her is as strong and full as ever. Her memory gives me courage to work hard, push beyond my comfort zone, be my best and most beautiful self, and to honor the amazing person she was.

Music, whether you are listening to it or playing it on an instrument, is both healing and empowering. Studies show that music can improve our attention span and help us build self-confidence, develop social skills, and give us a sense of belonging. According to a 2014 Wakefield Research survey of one thousand Americans age eighteen years and older, 86 percent said they preferred aural (listening) pleasures to visual ones in order to relax, with more than one-third choosing music as a way to help them decompress. In fact, music therapy is increasingly being used in neonatal units to soothe premature infants, as well as to treat depression in adults. Some hospitals have music piped into operating rooms to help surgeons relax.

In his book *Musicophilia*, Oliver Sacks writes eloquently about the power of music, which, he said, can "move us to the heights or depths of emotion." There are so many ways to listen to music these days, including streaming on your computer or smartphone, using an MP3 player, or turning on the radio in your car (music also helps to control road rage). There is no shortage of audio apps, such as iTunes, Spotify, and Pandora, which provide a traveling feast of music so you can tune out your stress.

Lift Your Voice (and Spirits) in Song. I wish I could carry a tune. Although I happen to love my own singing, I have a feeling if I sang aloud to my patients, the other Doris Day would show up and demand her name back! Sometimes I still try, and if it's in the right key I can almost get away with sounding good, but mostly I've learned to let it out when I'm alone and to lip-synch when I'm in public.

Singing, whether in public or in private, is unquestionably a wonderful way to relieve anxiety, especially if you're crooning upbeat music that puts you in a good mood. One of my favorites is "Happy" by Pharrell Williams, which puts smiles on so many faces. If you don't have the singing chops of Pharrell, but want to go vocal, stick to the shower or the karaoke machine. If you are able to carry a tune, join a choir (gospel or secular) or a community chorus (school, local theater company), or form a rock or hip-hop group. If you're really good, ask the manager of a local cabaret or coffeehouse if you can do a free set.

Release Your Inner Picasso. The mere act of creating art (without judgment about how good it is) can help us alleviate stress in many ways, and research shows that it also helps keep us young in mind and body. The Mayo Clinic recommended the benefits of painting and ceramics after conducting a four-year study that showed people who took up creative activities such as these in middle age were less likely to suffer memory loss.

My mom is a great artist and even now in her eighties continues to go to daily classes at the Art Students League in New York City to study her craft. She's won awards for her work and has the most amazing ability to adapt to new genres—from portraits to still lifes and watercolor to oil. I proudly have her work hanging in my office, and my children proudly hung her paintings in their dorm rooms when they were in college. They enjoy her artwork, and it brings them closer to her. Painting provides a distraction from everyday worries. If you've had a tiff with a colleague at work or you've had a disagreement with your spouse, get out a sketchpad and draw something to take your mind off what's making you anxious—even if it's just for a few minutes. After being engrossed in your sketches, you'll have a clearer head with which to tackle your problems. Adult coloring books are extremely popular because the activity creates a quality called "flow," which refers to being engaged in something that puts you in a meditative state where your mind is cleared of interfering thoughts. This artful flow has many of the same benefits of meditation, leaving you feeling more relaxed.

Dance Your Troubles Away. Lord Byron, the famous English Romantic poet, wrote, "On with the dance! Let joy be unconfined!" Anyone who has danced with abandon, be it at a club, at a wedding, or onstage, knows that it is a joyful experience. This is probably why dance has been a part of social and religious life throughout history in cultures around the world.

Dancing, or even just moving to a beat, can elevate your mood, not only because of the rhythmic movements but also because the physical activity releases endorphins (it's an exercise, after all). These hormones are your personal inner antidepressants. Plus, you'll also be listening to music, so you'll be getting the benefit of that proven relaxer at the same time. And it's worth noting that like music therapy, dance therapy is helping many people find their way out of emotional distress and move—literally—toward a serene way of life. When I was studying for my medical school exams, I would go to the gym for a run, have some dinner, and then sit at my desk and study relentlessly for hours. However, I was wise enough to take "dance breaks" to get my energy level back up and clear my mind for more studying. I would put on my favorite tunes and sing and dance my heart out. My favorite was Rick Astley's "Never Gonna Give You Up." I was then refreshed and ready to sit back down, happily out of breath, and study for another few hours before doing it again.

STEP SIX: "LAUGHTER IS THE SPARKLE OF THE SOUL" (ANCIENT PROVERB)

In biblical times, the wisdom that laughter is good for us was well known. As Proverbs 17:22 says: "A merry heart doeth good like a medicine; but a broken spirit drieth the bones." And, by extension, a broken spirit "drieth" your skin!

In fact, the Latin origin of the word *humor* means "fluid" or "moisture." Plus, you've probably heard that it takes more muscles to frown than to smile (not just an old wives' tale—it's true). Not only does your face look better when you smile, but a grin can alleviate the pain of an upsetting situation and improve your mood. According to one university study, humor associated with mirthful laughter (HAML) is a viable nonpharmacological practice that promotes greater health and wellness. HAML was also shown to help alleviate symptoms of a variety of chronic medical conditions.

Similarly, Dr. William E. Fry, a psychiatrist and emeritus associate clinical professor at Stanford University, reported an absence of the stress hormones called corticoids and catecholamines when people were engaged in laughter. Dr. Fry and his associates also showed that laughter boosts the immune system. About a decade ago, Dr. Madan Kataria burst out laughing for no apparent reason. Since then, he's helped to form more than three thousand Laughter Clubs throughout India, working toward the goal of creating millions of clubs around the world. In India, Laughter Clubs are now commonplace, and members meet on a daily basis in public parks or community centers. "When you laugh, you change," explains Kataria, whose fans include actors Goldie Hawn and John Cleese. "And when you change, the whole world changes around you." He could also have said, "When you laugh, the world laughs with you." On a recent trip to Thailand, I came across the laughing Buddha and it was my favorite of all the Buddhas I saw (see photo insert).

Like art and dance therapy, laughter therapy (also known as laughter yoga) can be practiced by anyone at any age. You can do laughing exercises in the privacy of your own home, but it's recommended that you laugh with others, as it is a great social and bonding experience— and it's contagious (in a good way). Laughing in a group will encourage you to lose your inhibitions. Laughter therapy exercises are simple to follow, and include pretending that someone just said something funny and letting out a hearty guffaw. Awkward at first, but it seems to work.

Laughing exercises the abdominal muscles, the joints, the spine, the diaphragm, and the muscles of the face. You take in four times as much oxygen while laughing than when you are sedentary and do not laugh. Your heart rate increases, and blood flows faster through your arteries. Chemical neurotransmitters produce painkilling and tranquilizing endorphins in the brain. Laughing can even burn calories (an added incentive for some).

STEP SEVEN: PAY IT FORWARD

Helping others is good for your mind, body, and spirit. A recent study by the University of North Carolina found that the type of happiness that comes from helping others and having a larger purpose in life produces more antibodies, which helps ward off illness. In addition to enhancing our immune system and making us happier, the social interaction that comes with volunteering can lower our heart rate and blood pressure, increase endorphin production, and shield against stress. I have been on the volunteer faculty of NYU Langone and attended the Tuesday morning dermatology clinic with the dermatology residents for twenty years. I get the opportunity to teach and supervise brilliant budding dermatologists as they treat patients who otherwise have little to no access to health care. I look forward to my Tuesday mornings because I somehow always learn more from the residents than I could possibly ever teach them. I also treat burn victims with lasers to help heal and erase their scars. I have one very special patient who had the sad experience of having her robe catch fire one morning while she was making breakfast for her family. She had burns over 50 percent of her body, going from the side of her face to her right arm, hand, breast, and back, making it difficult for her to raise her arm or hold hands. She drives two hours with her husband to come in for the treatments and she is so grateful for the care. It has been extremely special for me to watch her heal and recover her life. I received a letter from her, which I will cherish forever, and I will share it with you:

I recalled your exact words said to me when I first met you. During consultation, you recap what I discussed with you. You said to me that 'you are a very strong woman and I admire you.' You also said to me that I am to keep faith as, 'There is a light at the end of the tunnel.' I have been under your care for some time now due to the severe scarring of my upper right torso and neck. I must say that the 'tunnel light' you referred to has already appeared and is coming more into focus. As such, I am feeling much better about myself and so I must thank you sincerely from the bottom of my heart and keep up the good work you have engaged upon for all of us. Truer words have never been spoken as what you've said to me when we first met. My ultimate thanks to you and your professional staff who, in my opinion is second to none.

STEP EIGHT: COUNT YOUR BLESSINGS

Feeling happy with our lives starts with being grateful. The act of living in gratitude is the buffer that cushions us against our day-to-day struggles and pain. If you are grateful for all that you have and all that you've been given, it is difficult to encounter an obstacle you cannot deal with. Gratitude is what keeps us from falling into a pit of despair when bad stuff happens to us. We all have our struggles, and we all experience pain at some point in our lives. But no matter how bad things seem at the time, we can always find something to be grateful for. If you are in good health, you should be grateful for that, because being healthy in mind and body is the foundation on which everything else is built. Once you become aware of the little gifts that come your way every day, you will find that you notice more and more of life's everyday miracles. I'm not saying that you will always have a good day, but noticing the good things that happen will help offset the negative things.

After the loss of my sister I went through so much, and one day I realized that I had a choice: I could make something good out of everything, even if there was no good in it at all. From that day forward I found so much to be grateful for and so much I could do to help others as part of healing myself. I miss my sister just as much, but I'm able to channel that energy and convert it into something productive rather than drowning in the pain.

I know with every fiber of my being that being a physician is a privilege and an honor. I am grateful to be able to do what I do every day, and every day I wake up excited to learn more and continue to hone my skills. At the end of each day's work I have a sense of euphoria from the experience of seeing patients; I love having an impact on their health and well-being, and I love seeing them experience more hope and control over their lives. I don't take a minute of my life for granted; I have seen and experienced too much to think that I have time for that. I know this is my one life; I don't get to do it over. But I want to live life in such a way that I'd want to repeat it over and over again if I could.

I am grateful for my husband of nearly thirty years and my children, who give me so much joy and who are people I admire and respect and love spending time with. They are my best friends and they have my heart. My mom is alive and thriving, showing incredible resillience after recently losing her husband of more than fifty years. She is an incredible artist, and to this day she takes care of me instead of my having to worry about and take care of her. I encourage you to find a path where you can feel the same, to live as if this is the only day there is. If you're lucky you'll get countless days to practice this again and again. Keep working on your path until every day is that day.

STEP NINE: SAVOR THE MOMENT

It's 10 p.m., but my children, Andrew, age three, and Sabrina, age five, are still up. They rush to open the door. "Mommy, Mommy!" Big hugs and kisses are followed by priceless cuddle time and a book before bed. A few evenings later it's the same scenario; but this time, racked with guilt about coming home late so often, I bring them each a little treat. Their joy at seeing me shifts to excitement over what I brought, and my guilt is relieved by the bribe gift. The next time, no hugs, just a search for what I had brought, and tears in Andrew's eyes. "That's all you brought?" That's when it hit me that the gift they really needed was me. Nothing material could ever match the open arms and love of a mother coming home, no matter how late. Another evening Sabrina, then six, sees me putting on my coat and asks where I'm going. "To a meeting," I tell her as smoothly as I can. Her big, brown, innocent eyes look into mine. "Mommy, don't go to the meeting. Stay home and take care of your family." I kiss her and, holding back tears, go off to the meeting required of all residents. The pain of that time echoes with renewed sharpness even today, as our daughter, now seventeen, begins her college search. I know I will soon be the one wishing she would come home.

Those early years of motherhood were tough and in many ways self-inflicted, because the day after I graduated I started my own practice, with no business background, in a crowded zip code on New York's Upper East Side. At first, a difficult patient or staff issue would consume me. While our dinner conversation flowed, my mind was still back in the office. Then one day I realized I had to change. That was the day I watched in horror as our young daughter exploded at my husband and me, her arms flailing, mirroring my behavior when I would come home stressed and yell at everyone over the slightest thing. Mini Me. Resolving not to impose my professional worries of the day on my family, I committed to compartmentalizing. Separating work and home would enable me to be 100 percent in the moment. Over time, my resolution and my deeper experience with life and work have given me a better sense of control and comfort. There will never be enough time in the day to do all the things I want to do, but reminding myself that this is the path I've chosen in my life and I'm going to make it the right path helps immensely. I have been fortunate to have a loving and patient husband, parents who lived in our building and were able to frequently pitch in, and wonderful role models and friends to help support and guide me. They have shown me that balance is truly a state of mind.

Now it's your turn: Let this simple exercise be your first step toward greater balance and happiness in your own life. Create a note in your phone or journal—someplace you often look and will be reminded— and list small changes you would like to make and the desired results. For every goal you list, from separating work and family time to taking quiet moments for yourself, also list the reason. This is important, because being conscious of *why* you wish to make change and *what* you want to achieve will fuel your journey.

(Sample)

Things to Change	Why?	Results
Separate work and home life.	*Put less stress on family.*	*Balance!*

STEP TEN: MINDFUL EATING

Mindful eating means being aware of what's going into your body, which affects every organ, including your skin, both directly and indirectly. You may think that as long as you are using an expensive skin cream with a bunch of natural-sounding ingredients and scientific names, your skin will be properly nourished. Not true. While a great skin care regimen is essential, it will never replace proper skin nutrition that comes from within. I can assure you that good nutrition will help you toward your goal of having healthy and youthful skin. Here are a few tips that will benefit your skin while satisfying your body and soul.

Eat Raw Fruits and Vegetables. Fruits and vegetables are a superior source of skin-enhancing nutrients, including antioxidants, and you'll really reap their benefits if you avoid cooking away much of what nature put into that apple, carrot, or bowl of blueberries. Remember also that the skins of many fruits and veggies, such as apples, pears, and tomatoes, are chock-full of nutrients and give you much-needed fiber. There's nothing wrong with indulging in healthy smoothies now and then, but whenever possible, eat a whole fruit. By the same token, it is wonderful to steam your veggies to go with a hot meal or cook tomatoes to make a sauce, but be sure to also munch on fresh raw cauliflower, broccoli, carrots, spinach, and grape tomatoes for lunch and for snacks. Broccoli contains a high amount of isothiocyanates, an excellent cancer-fighting compound.*

The easiest way to think of it is that isothiocyanates work by turning on cancer-fighting genes and turning off others that feed on the disease. Kale, spinach, Swiss chard, beet greens, and other vegetables provide important nutrients to support bone health, eye health, and even prevent cancer. Spirulina provides high levels of antioxidants, including polyphenols. This superantioxidant is a powerhouse weapon against premature aging. A study published by Tufts University showed that anthocyanins (the pigments that give them their deep color) in blueberries appear to combat oxidative stress. Oxidative stress is one of the main causes of aging. Anthocyanins also aid your brain in the production of dopamine, a chemical that is critical to coordination, memory function, and your mood. Your skin and figure will thank you!

Keep Your Skin Hydrated. When skin is well hydrated, it is more plump and resilient. This is due, at least in part, to an ingredient in the skin called hyaluronic acid. As I've mentioned, the job of hyaluronic acid is to hold water in the skin. When there is adequate water

---

* *Source:* Sheetal Gupta and Jamuna Prakash, "Studies on Indian Green Leafy Vegetables for Their Antioxidant Activity," *Plant Foods for Human Nutrition* 64, no. 1 (2009): 39–45.

from inside and outside, the skin looks healthier and more vibrant and is less prone to wrinkles, so drink lots of fluids throughout the day. You've probably heard the six to eight glasses of water a day as a reasonable rule of thumb, but you may need more or less depending on your activity level. Also, try to control your salt intake, because even with normal blood pressure, an excess of salt in the diet will lead to water retention, which can make your skin, especially around the eyes, puffier. Too little salt is as bad as too much, so if you are an avid exerciser and you sweat a lot, you may have to add salt to your diet. Be sure to use iodized salt to assure that you don't become iodine-deficient. Two of my favorite drinks are naturally sparkling water (not seltzer), with a twist of lemon or lime, and green tea as part of my daily fluid intake. I also like to make a large pitcher of water, adding lemon, lime, orange, or cucumber slices, and let them "marinate" overnight. The water will have a refreshing flavor without being sweet. I can easily go through a pitcher a day, sometimes refilling several times. You can also eat your water. Foods like cucumber, lettuce, and watermelon are packed with water and also have a low glycemic index and fiber, which gives them added value.

Avoid Simple Sugars. Simple sugars like table sugar and refined carbohydrates are bad for your skin, just as they are bad for the rest of your body. They are empty calories. If you fill up on them, you are depriving yourself of food with skin-boosting nutrients. Also, if you eat too much food containing simple sugars and other simple carbs, or foods with a high glycemic index (also known as blood sugar levels), you increase your risk of weight gain, contracting type 2 diabetes and other health problems, and lowering your energy. All of this will also contribute to unhealthy, prematurely aging skin.

Avoid Soda. All sodas, even diet sodas, contain phosphates, or phosphoric acid, a weak acid that can lead to heart and kidney problems including kidney stones, muscle loss, and osteoporosis, and may also trigger accelerated aging. If you have to have soda, at least try to avoid caramelized soda such as colas and opt instead for the clear versions, as those tend to contain less of the acids that have a negative impact on your health.

Eat Fiber-Rich Foods. Fiber reduces the risk of many health diseases and conditions, including heart disease, diabetes, obesity, colon cancer, and hemorrhoids. It also makes for good digestion and elimination, which help to keep your skin looking vibrant. By some estimates, the average American eats only about one-third of the amount of fiber needed daily for peak health. Be sure to include whole grains, especially bran, in your diet every day, and eat fruits whole.

Indulge, but Don't Overdo It. Mindful eating means being more in tune with your body so you can make choices that are right for you. Your metabolism will adjust to those ups and downs. Listen to your body; take small bites; chew your food well so you can savor the flavor; don't read, use your phone, or watch TV while you eat; and stop when you're full. It's okay to indulge once in a while in your favorite treat, whether it's chocolate (preferably dark), ice cream, or whatever your guilty pleasure, but remember, a "treat" is a once-in-a-while food, not an everyday staple. If you allow yourself to indulge every now and then, even if it's a fatty or salty snack such as potato chips and pretzels, you won't feel deprived. But making poor food choices on a regular basis and overindulging will do in you and your skin!

Experiment in the Kitchen. I love to cook and experiment with recipes I've collected, and I encourage you to do the same. I am constantly modifying recipes by reducing the amount of skin-damaging salt, using healthful alternatives to butter, and amping up the flavor and aroma by adding spices and herbs. Right now you may feel that you simply don't have time to cook, but once you get started, you'll realize that spending a little time in the kitchen will go a long way toward easing tension and tapping into your creative spirit! Resist that urge to go to the fast-food joint to pick up dinner on your way home, and put down that phone if you were planning to call in for pizza.

If you opt for delivery, try the healthier preportioned fare that comes in a box from companies such as Blue Apron, HelloFresh, and Freshly. Freshly stands out as a new company that makes eating healthy easier than ever by working as both your "personal chef and nutritionist." They do the work for you, from ingredient sourcing to recipe creation to cooking, and deliver fresh, gourmet ready-made meals designed to help you optimize your health. Each meal is carefully curated with all-natural ingredients and packaged using the most advanced technology to ensure your food stays fresh. No grocery shopping, cooking, or cleaning—all you have to do is heat and enjoy.

The meals are prepared with:

- no artificial ingredients;

- no hydrogenated oils; and

- no refined sugars.

ASK DR. DAY

Q: *I'm in my thirties and I have a wicked sweet tooth. I don't go a day without eating a dessert or treat. I've heard that sugar can age my skin. Is that true?*

DD: The answer is yes. Glycation occurs due to a variety of factors, including genetics, sun exposure, hormones, cigarette smoke, pollution, stress, and foods.

Glycation is the reaction between sugar and protein, like collagen residues. It leads to the formation of abnormal products called AGEs (advanced glycation end products), which are toxic for the cells. Cross-linking of collagen results in increased stiffening of the skin and then wrinkle formation.

While glycation occurs naturally in the skin over time, there is an acceleration of the process in sun-exposed skin. Studies show that there may be some protection against skin damage with a higher intake of vegetables, olive oil, fish, and legumes, and a lower intake of butter, margarine, and other milk products, and sugar products. Of the factors of aging leading to glycation, sun exposure is higher on the list than sugars, but hold the sugar and don't forget the sunscreen.

There are also ingredients to help protect against AGEs, including L-carnosine (amino peptide), which is a natural body product. Our body's nerve cells and muscle cells contain naturally high levels of L-carnosine; *however*, the level of L-carnosine decreases with age, so we need to look for it in foods and supplements.

Another important category of ingredients is adaptogens. These moderate the stress response, strengthen the body's immune system, and improve resistance at the cellular level, thereby prolonging the onset of fatigue, exhaustion, injury, and/or illness. Some well-known adaptogens include ginseng, rosemary, holy basil, ashwagandha, ginseng or rhodiola, Schisandra, and aloe vera.

Samantha Heller, registered dietitian, senior clinical nutritionist at NYU Langone, radio host, and author of *The Only Cleanse*, weighs in on nutrition and the skin-diet connection:

Q: *How does proper nutrition help the skin?*
SH: Everything you eat becomes part of the tapestry and fabric of your body. We might eat a banana and think, "*That tastes good*," then forget about it, but your body is rendering that banana into tiny molecules that get incorporated into your skin and other organs. Those molecules will affect your body's ability

to function in either a positive or a negative way. The food we eat is transferred to the skin to support it (or not), depending on what we eat.

Q: What are some of the best foods and nutrients for the skin?
SH: Healthy fats, such as omega-3 fatty acids, are fantastic for the skin. They help reduce inflammation and resist the effects of ultraviolet rays from the sun. One of the biggest aging issues for the skin is oxidative stress, and omega-3s help reduce the oxidative stress and slow down the aging process. Fish is the richest source of omega-3s, but there is some concern now about mercury, dioxin, and PCBs in fish.

There are alternative sources of omega-3 fatty acids, including walnuts, tofu, flaxseed, and purslane, which is a weed that grows in my backyard (you can get it in health food stores). Avocado, olive oil, and nuts are also great sources of unsaturated fats, which are good for your skin, your immune system, and your nervous system.

Q: There have been some reports that say soy isn't good for you. What's the latest?
SH: All the bad news about soy is a myth. I have breast cancer survivor patients eating tofu and edamame and drinking soy milk. It's also safe for men. People have been eating tofu for five thousand years with no ill effects. There is preliminary research that suggests soy might even decrease some symptoms of menopause, although this is not the case for everyone.

Q: What are carotenoids?
SH: Carotenoids are fantastically healthy compounds that give fruits and vegetables their bright colors. Carrots are bright orange because they contain a carotenoid called beta-carotene. Beta-carotene is one of more than five hundred carotenoids

found in nature. Carotenoids act as strong antioxidants that protect the skin against photodamage and UV rays. They also stimulate immune response and guard against some types of cancers. You want to eat oranges, sweet potatoes, carrots, butternut squashes, kale, and broccoli, all of which are great foods for your skin. Broccoli also contains a high amount of isothiocyanates, which work by turning on cancer-fighting genes and turning off others that feed on the disease.

Q: *What's your opinion on gluten-free foods?*

SH: The only reason to be on a gluten-free diet is if you have celiac disease or you have a non-celiac gluten intolerance or other medical reason to avoid eating gluten. Other than that, there is no reason to avoid gluten. For most people, eating wheat, barley, or rice is fine.

Q: *How important are vitamins C and E for the skin?*

SH: Vitamin C is critical for collagen synthesis and acts as scaffolding for the skin, so we need that in our diet. It's a powerful antioxidant and it works closely with vitamin E. It helps protect against the sun and you need adequate amounts of vitamin C and zinc for wound healing.

STEP ELEVEN: THE SKIN-NY ON SEX (AND ORGASMS)

If your face has lost its healthy radiance, consider going for "The Big O Glow." Whether you have a spouse, partner, or you're single, studies show that physical contact can help lower our stress levels that can cause us to age more rapidly. Even hugging or cuddling can reduce blood pressure, and kissing releases chemicals that are known to eliminate stress hormones.

Studies show that orgasms occur through a direct connection to the brain through the vagus nerve rather than going through the typical network of nerves through the spinal cord. The vagus nerve is the longest cranial nerve, it has motor and sensory fibers and, because it passes through the neck and chest to the abdomen, has the widest distribution in the body. The result of an orgasm is release of endorphins, which are neurotransmitters that promote a sense of overall well-being, and oxytocin, also known as the "feel good hormone." At the same time, our levels of cortisol, the stress hormone, lower, which produces a winning hormonal cocktail for pleasure and contentment.

Sex or masturbation can also give our immune system a boost. Having an orgasm once or twice a week will also increase your production of the immune-strengthening antibody immunoglobulin by a third.

Other facts about sex, orgasms, and our skin:

I often tell my patients that sex three times a week is the secret to a happy marriage and it turns out that there's science to back that up. A Scottish study found that loving, supportive couples who had intercourse three or more times a week appeared on average ten years younger than their actual age. Healthy, happy, and younger—now there's a perfect example of Beyond Beautiful!

Sex and masturbation are also great ways for insomniacs to get their sleep fix, as they are said to release endorphins and provide a better night's sleep—another factor that helps get rid of those tired, baggy eyes.

Good sex is also good for a woman's health. According to a 2016 Michigan State University study of more than 2,200 people age fifty-seven and older, women who reported the most satisfying sex had a lower risk for high blood pressure and other cardiovascular conditions than women who had either mediocre sex or no sex. It seems women's hearts just might grow stronger from the hormones produced during orgasms.

Take Paula, who had been seeing me regularly for skin cancer checkups. She was a widow in her mid-fifties. Her husband, to whom she had been happily married for over twenty years, had died of prostate cancer two years earlier, and she really missed him. She told me wonderful stories about their years together and I could see her eyes light up when she spoke of him.

She also expressed she was lonely and wanted treatments to help her look more "refreshed" so she might meet someone new: Years had gone by without her finding another partner or husband. She confessed that she didn't feel very pretty anywhere, even "down there," and that she had issues with vaginal dryness but did not want to take any hormones. I created an aesthetic blueprint for her and we started on her journey to rejuvenation, including a relatively new set of treatments for nonsurgically rejuvenating the vaginal area using fractional ablative lasers like the CO2 laser, the non-ablative Fotona laser, or using radio-frequency energy. The results are often dramatic with improved lubrication, enhanced orgasm, decreased incontinence, and a more beautiful vagina. Women want to feel beautiful everywhere, and now they can! The treatments are virtually painless, and while a series of three-to-five treatments is usually recommended, you can see improvement in as little as one treatment.

Paula, who was so happy with the treatments, had still yet to start dating when it was time for a little extracurricular advice. I said until she was ready to let someone into her life (and bed), she should visit a shop in town that discreetly sold sex toys. (You can also purchase these intimate items online at www.evesgarden.com.)

At her next follow-up a few months later, as soon as I walked into the room I could see that her skin had a rosy glow. I said, "You did what I suggested, didn't you?" and she nodded, surprised that I could see the difference in her. And we both giggled like schoolgirls. Not long after that, she told me that she had a boyfriend and the relationship was getting serious.

Sometimes you've got to figure out how to please yourself before you can open up and meet someone new!

Here's what Palm Springs, California–based sex coach Laura Anne Rowell told me in an interview:

Q: *So "afterglow" is a real facial phenomenon?*
LAR: That blush we get after sex is the collagen and the estrogen being released. It gives us a sense of fulfillment, completeness, and general well-being. It can last anywhere from one hour to several days. There are even blushes called "After Glow" and "Glow 'Gasm" that try to re-create that healthy flush, which happens when oxygen flows into the capillaries, usually after vigorous sex.

Q: *Why does sex make us look better?*
LAR: People with active sex lives tend to exude more confidence. That shows in their face. When we have sex with someone who appreciates our body, it makes us feel more beautiful. In my couples workshops I teach something called the "eye gaze" that releases oxytocin hormones. It actually reduces the craving for drugs and alcohol, which are bad for the skin. There is a kind of meditative state that occurs when you make sustained eye contact with someone. You can just lie in bed side by side and stare into each other's eyes for a few minutes. It's even more intimate than actual sex. It's a part of Tantric sex, which I recommend to everyone. It involves sitting with your partner and looking into their eyes.

I have another game I call "Kitten Play," where you just touch someone on different parts of the body, like the chest, legs, and face, to see how your partner and then you respond. I call it "Kitten Play" because a kitten will show you where it wants to be stroked. If you're really present and in the moment your body will react to this touching. You can touch the genital area, but don't focus on it, because it's more about foreplay.

Q: *How important is an orgasm?*

LAR: Sex is different than an orgasm. Having an orgasm gives you a feeling of euphoria and helps lower stress by lowering levels of cortisol. I believe orgasms should be as much a part of your daily routine as brushing your teeth. We all have stressful lives—why not fit a daily orgasm into your routine? It helps you sleep better, frees up your mind, and closes down the part of the brain that has the functions of anxiety, stress, and fear.

Q: *How do you help women who don't feel attractive or have a negative body image that prevents them from enjoying sex?*

LAR: I learned that when you reach a certain age, you just don't care anymore about looking like a twenty-year-old. Older women who are still sexually active have more youthful-looking skin in part because they feel desired. I'm in my forties and I've gained weight, which many women in middle age do, and there was a point when I felt bad about not being a size 2 anymore. I tried webcam modeling as research and to put myself out there. I was amazed at how many women my age were gorgeous! I remember what I was like in my twenties, and I miss my body from back then, but my mind is so much better now. I know so much more, and I have a better imagination so I can experience more. There's something about different body shapes and sizes that's erotic. As we get older, our bodies change, but we should appreciate being voluptuous. Look at your body with gratitude as something that has gone on a wonderful journey and has given you so much. Any procedure you decide to get, do it for yourself and not for anyone else!

Q: *What do you say to women who are not in the mood for sex?*

LAR: I'd ask them what the cause is for their not feeling sexy. If they are in a relationship, I would want to find out if there is something that their partner isn't doing, or is doing to make them feel bad, or is it something in themselves. I have a client who is a doctor with beautiful red hair that she wears back in a ponytail all the time. She's a tomboy, which is fine, and she told me that it's easier for her to wear her hair back at work. I tell women like her to take some time to make yourself feel more attractive. Let your hair down, literally and figuratively! Do it for yourself—never for anyone else. Make yourself feel pretty. Don't wear those sweatpants when you get home, even if you live alone. Put on a sexy nightgown for yourself. Take a bubble bath. I understand we all have busy lives, but put on a pretty lacy bra under your uniform.

Coming up…discover the best skin care regimen to use from your twenties to your sixties and beyond. Everyone deserves to look the best they can, for whatever decade they're living in.

CHAPTER TEN

Beyond Beautiful Through the Ages

Your Daily, Weekly, and Monthly Maintenance Plan (Plus Other Tips)

"You can be gorgeous at thirty, charming at forty, and irresistible for the rest of your life."

—*Coco Chanel*

By now you're practically an honorary dermatologist, medical detective, and master of understanding the powerful mind connection with your skin and body. In this chapter I've broken down my recommended beauty routines for each decade, from your twenties to your sixties and beyond, based on the changes that occur on every level of your skin.

We have a different kind of beauty in our twenties than we do in our fifties, and I'll tell you what the things you see on the surface during those decades mean on a deeper level, and what you can do about them at home and with your aesthetic dermatologist. Prepare to go skin diving!

Let's start with the basic skin care regimen that you can use throughout life, starting in your twenties.

THE ROARING TWENTIES

> "Everyone goes on about how hard it is to be a teenager, but actually I think it's tougher to be in your twenties because you're expected to be a grown-up and expected to earn your own living and be successful, and I think you feel like a kid still."
> —*Nigel Cole, English film and TV director*

In your twenties you have the natural beauty of youth. Your skin is still plump and firm, the sun and life's stressors have not yet left their mark. Patients I see in this age-group are usually coming in for treatments either to look more attractive, which is different than more beautiful, or to stay ahead of the aging process by learning about preventive treatments.

Millennials and Gen Xers will take an average of 25,700 selfies in their lifetime. It's an age of online everything, with choreographed and curated posts adapted to the particular site—a sultry look for Tinder, professional profile for LinkedIn, perfectly composed and airbrushed shots for Instagram, and family-friendly posts for Facebook since their parents are also posting these days.

The twenties are a time of great opportunity and also great uncertainty. For the first time in decades the kids don't expect to do as well as their parents, and they are channeling that into more adventure and living for the moment. They pay attention to appearance and are more willing to try new products and procedures than their parents were at their age.

People in their twenties will often try a treatment or have a procedure like fillers for the lips to make them bigger, sexier, and more attractive, or Botox Cosmetic to freeze the forehead to prevent lines or signs of aging, even though they bake in the sun. They may visit a spa for a laser treatment or an injection rather than see a trained aesthetic physician, because the treatments are seen as temporary and interchangeable, like an outfit or hair color, when in reality they are anything but that.

In fact, the fillers and other treatments I discuss in this book, while theoretically "temporary" in that FDA indications say they last one to two years, depending on the product, often last much longer; and, more importantly, they change the way we see ourselves. Also, depending on how much product is used, especially in areas such as the lips, breasts, and buttocks, they may cause permanent changes in the skin, causing it to stretch beyond its ability to return to its original form. This is no longer a matter of aging gracefully, but rather of changing features. It's not always safe and not always a good idea. This is the best age to see your aesthetic dermatologist to come up with your aesthetic blueprint, or, your plan to help yourself age beautifully and gracefully. It does not mean having treatments or surgery, it means understanding what you can do for your skin to protect it so it always looks its best. What you do now, for good or bad, will show decades later when it's too late to take it back.

I find that in most cases, *no* is more often a better answer than *yes*. It takes discussion and effort to guide my patients through this decade, to help them see their beauty, and to seek true age prevention rather than to change how they look.

Another concern that starts in the twenties is uneven skin tone, which often comes from a combination of being on hormonal contraception (birth control pills), usually for five years or longer, combined with sun exposure. The condition is called melasma. If you have melasma, you need to be extra vigilant about sun protection and also any treatments that create heat in the skin, including lasers and intense pulsed light. There are excellent treatments your dermatologist can provide, and also medications including ingredients such as hydroquinone, azelaic acid, and tranexamic acid. I also use oral over-the-counter and prescription supplements such as GliSODin skin brightening supplement and oral tranexamic acid.

The good news is that in your twenties you don't need a ten-step skin care routine, and you can find nearly everything you do need right at your local drugstore. It is important, though, to get into the routine of taking great care of your skin. I call this aesthetic hygiene: it's getting in the habit and creating an innate discipline to take great care of your skin, so you will already be protecting it from damage as you get older, and your chronological age will just be a number and your biologic age will be much younger.

Having great skin when you're in your twenties is a lot about lifestyle, so if you're drinking too much, working long hours, grabbing food on the run, and staying out too late, it will show in your glow (or the lack of it). Getting enough sleep, eating healthfully, and keeping your stress levels in check will help your skin stay fresh and vibrant.

That said, your twenties are also about being preventive, because good habits now mean better skin later on. My hope is you'll decide to perfect your pale instead of seeking a tan. If you feel strongly that a tan is what you want, I would steer you to sunless tanners and bronzers. These have come a long way. Some of my favorites include: St. Tropez sunless tanner and Clarins Radiance-Plus Golden Glow Booster.

Daily

Use a moisturizer with SPF: Your twenties are all about prevention. Not all prevention is the same: everyone needs sunscreen for prevention of aging, but not everyone needs Botox for prevention. Sunscreen will literally save your skin. It is your first line of defense against UV damage, which accelerates the aging of your skin. The fact is that UV rays, both UVA and UVB, are the culprit behind 80 percent of the visible signs of aging. Wearing SPF 30 and above sunscreen daily will help prevent skin cancer. I see the worst sunburns occur on cloudy days and the most sun damage in runners who exercise and train outdoors.

I always say, "Skin cancer doesn't care how fit and healthy you are." And know this: even if you do use sunscreen and you find that you somehow got a tan, the tan still counts and may lead to skin cancer and premature aging. It might take ten or more years to show, but after twenty years in practice, I hear over and over from my patients: "I wish I had used more sunscreen when I was younger." Your fifty-year-old self is pleading with you to please be sun-smart in your twenties.

This means:

- Avoid midday sun when possible.

- Stay in the shade when you can.

- Wear sun protective clothing.

- Apply sunscreen with an SPF of 30 or higher and reapply every two hours.

- Wear sunglasses and a hat. (Look for larger sunglasses that protect the delicate area of skin around your eyes. Wearing UVA/UVB-protective sunglasses also helps delay or prevent cataracts.)

- Use an over-the-counter retinol: Collagen can start to break down as early as your mid-twenties. After the age of twenty, 1 percent less collagen is produced in the dermis each year. Using an over-the-counter retinol like Roc Retinol Night Cream, Neutrogena Rapid Wrinkle Repair, or Olay Regenerist Intensive Repair Treatment before you go to bed can help stave off the signs of aging. Retinoids not only stimulate collagen production, but they also help even out skin tone, making your face a perfect, smooth, clear palate onto which you can apply some head-turning makeup (you can apply it right up to the lower lash line, but be careful not to get any in your eyes).

Another major myth I hear day in and day out is that retinol makes you more sun-sensitive. The reality is that most retinol products will be deactivated and made less effective by the sun. Having retinol on your skin does not make you more sun-sensitive. The other misconception is that retinol will thin out your skin. Also not true. Retinol helps to strengthen and improve the collagen layer of your skin, which makes your skin thicker and younger; but it does normalize and flatten the outer layer of your skin, which makes your skin smoother and less wrinkled over time. For some with very fair skin, that can make them slightly more sun-sensitive.

A young woman in her twenties came in for a follow-up recently, and she was very upset because her facialist insisted that the retinol I recommended was thinning her skin. Beware of "spa science"! Be sure to see only a dermatologist for skin care advice and guidance and to learn the science of evidence-based medicine.

Weekly

Exfoliate your face and body. You should exfoliate weekly because skin cells may be slower to naturally slough off as you age and your skin gets drier. This leaves it looking dull and can accentuate wrinkles. I often recommend exfoliating more gently but more often, using a glycolic over salicylic acid in a lower concentration. I also like cleansing cloths that are pre-moistened and can be used with or without water; they are also available in gently exfoliating form.

Monthly

Cleanse all makeup brushes and hairbrushes. Soak them for at least fifteen minutes in baby shampoo and rinse with lukewarm water.

BONUS PROCEDURES

I see more and more women in their twenties asking about "preventive" aesthetic procedures, such as:

Clear + Brilliant Laser: This gentle laser results in very little downtime and helps to even out skin tone and improve skin texture. Treatments should be given in a series at intervals of two to four weeks. Be sure to not have a suntan...ever...but especially not when having any laser treatment.

Microdermabrasion: This uses crystals gently blasted at the skin and then vacuumed back up to help exfoliate, clean out pores, even out tone, and remove the dead outer layer to leave your skin smooth and soft.

Chemical peels consisting of glycolic and/or salicylic acid: These can be irritating and should not be done if you have a tan or are about to have sun exposure. These peels come in many different concentrations and combinations and can be very effective in improving skin tone and texture and removing dark spots, as well as in treating skin conditions like acne and even rosacea.

Isolaz deep pore cleansing: Photopneumatic energy helps clear out the pores, followed by intense pulsed light to kill acne-causing bacteria and also reduce redness and chances of scarring. This is great for those with acne persisting into the twenties or those starting to get adult acne.

Laser hair removal: This is a great decade to get rid of unwanted hair. Results are long-lasting and make it possible to get rid of the hair and visits for waxing. For those who get regular ingrown hairs, this is an excellent option. When the follicle is gone, as it is after laser hair removal, there's no hair or follicle to be ingrown. It works best in those who have darker hair and lighter skin, but many lasers now treat a broad range of skin types.

THE THRILLING THIRTIES

"Time and tide wait for no man, but time always stands still for a woman of thirty."

—*Robert Frost*

Thirty is typically the age when women are moving up in their careers, and when they begin, or have begun, to think about marriage or settling down with a partner. Many are also having children (if they're not already moms). The thirties is definitely a time to start thinking about antiaging products as you realize you're not immortal, and you are at risk of turning into your mother if you don't take care of your skin (and this is true even if you adore your mom!). The natural aging process usually begins in the late twenties and early thirties when the production of collagen starts to decrease, leading to thinner and more lax skin. There is also diminished functioning of the sweat and oil glands, making the skin drier. I start to see more patients with rosacea, which is often confused with acne (see page 154 of chapter 8, "Don't Be Rash"). Other changes I see in the thirties are blotchy discolorations on the face and chest, early signs of volume loss in the midface, and deepening of fine lines between and around the eyes.

Hormonal flare-ups and cystic, stress-related pimples often plague thirty-somethings as well. Products containing caffeine, peptides, vitamin C, and antioxidants can make a big difference during this decade. It's important to try to get enough sleep and stay hydrated by drinking lots of water. In addition to the daily SPF, consider adding the following to your skin care routine.

Daily

Use an antioxidant serum. Antioxidants are key to your beauty routine once you hit age thirty. Antioxidants act like extinguishers to help put out any fires caused by UV rays. Let's face it, we don't always remember to apply and reapply sunscreen. Given these lapses, serums with vitamin C, vitamin E, and ferulic acid help repair the skin during the day. It's the best time to see your dermatologist for a skin care routine that is at the cosmeceutical level, used alone, or in combination with drugstore products, before layering on your sunscreen every day.

Use a prescription- or cosmeceutical-strength retinol. While twenty-somethings can get away with OTC retinols, now is the time to consider asking your dermatologist for a cosmeceutical-strength retinol to use at night. These are often stronger and combined with other ingredients to give them extra strength without extra irritation. Don't forget to apply on your neck and décolletage (two places that show early signs of aging).

It's time to pay special attention to the eye area by using a daily cream. Don't rub! Pat on an eye cream with key ingredients like retinol, niacinamide, and caffeine. There are also eye cream products with vitamin C, which is excellent for brightening.

Several Times a Week

A few times a week, try an exfoliating alpha hydroxy acid (AHA) product: Once you hit your thirties, there are many things going on beneath the surface that you can't see. Deep within your skin's layers, the dermis loses support and the skin become less bouncy. On the epidermis, the outermost surface layers, cellular renewal slows and your skin appears discolored and duller. To combat these visible changes, you can add an AHA product to your regimen two or three times a week. An alpha hydroxy acid helps prevent the buildup of dead skin cells, minimizes pores, and evens out skin texture and tone.

Monthly

A monthly cleanser or peel with salicylic or lactic acid will help brighten uneven texture and clear up breakouts (as I said earlier, acne isn't just for teenagers).

Bonus Treatments

Fraxel 1927 Laser: This laser reduces sun damage. Treatments should be done in a series, at one-month intervals, and not when you have a tan, but by now you know you should never have a tan! After the treatment, your skin will feel hot for about half an hour, will be red for a few hours, and then flaky for about five to seven days. You can wear makeup the day after. This treatment leaves your skin feeling soft and smooth and helps eliminate sun damage, which lowers your risk of skin cancer.

Isolaz: This office treatment uses photopneumatic energy for non-traumatic deep pore cleansing and improvement of skin texture and tone. It also helps to improve acne scars and reduces redness.

Fotona: This is a powerful combination of Erbium and Nd:YAG lasers, which work to tighten and resurface the skin. The depth ranges from light to deep, depending on the settings your doctor chooses. This laser is also great for getting rid of sebaceous hyperplasia, those pesky overgrown oil glands that can leave your skin looking bumpy, and for treating brown/sun spots as well. Depending on the settings and hand pieces used, the Fotona will aid in skin tightening and reducing unwanted fat on the body.

Neuromodulators: The early signs of lines that are beginning to remain after you've made certain expressions will respond to neuromodulators. This is considered preventive treatment and will help retrain your muscles to make more positive expressions and to maintain symmetry as you age.

Fillers: This may be the time to consider an hyaluronic acid (HA) filler to help treat the early signs of volume loss in the midface and chin area and to help maintain and enhance your beauty without changing it.

THE FLAUNT-IT FORTIES

"I'm not forty; I'm eighteen with twenty-two years' experience."
—*Anonymous*

The forties are such a fun decade in life because we are not just wiser, we are sexier! I was so dreading turning forty, and I really didn't take my fortieth birthday well at all. For some reason, from a very young age, I made up my mind that forty was far enough away that I could safely consider it as "old." All my patients and friends in their fifties told me how much they loved their forties and what a wonderful decade it was. It took some work to get past my old mind-set, but I did, and I have to agree my forties were fantastic! What I realized when I hit forty myself was that I was still young but I also had experience.

One aspect of the latter part of the forties is that most women enter perimenopause (the phase right before menopause begins), which means the body goes into a hormonal flux that can affect our mood and our skin. The collagen and elastin fibers break and clump and the skin loses elasticity, which causes wrinkles and folds. At this point women often see their skin start to sag, even if it's not visible to the rest of the world. It's also a time to consider seeing your aesthetic dermatologist to develop a personal aesthetic blueprint, which is your road map to keeping you looking your best and avoiding the need for surgery. My strategy has been to start younger with smaller procedures, rather than to wait and ultimately need greater intervention later on. What you do at home is just as important; while you still need to use antioxidants and SPF in the morning, try incorporating the following into your routine as well.

Daily

I recommend using a peptide- and growth factor–based serum daily. Peptides are protein fragments composed of amino acids that act like building blocks of the skin. They send messages telling your skin to do a specific job such as to stimulate collagen. By applying a serum daily, you will help to combat the expression lines that come from decades of smiling, laughing, or, for some, grimacing.

In your forties, adding an eye cream is a good idea. The eyes are generally one of the first places to show signs of aging because the skin is super delicate in that region. Look for an emollient formula that has antioxidants or retinol to see the best results. Try adding an eye serum under your nightly moisturizer.

Switch to a retinol combined with antiaging ingredients. This is the time to talk to your dermatologist about cosmeceutical-strength retinoids that are buoyed by antiaging ingredients for greater efficacy. I like Skin Better AlphaRet, SkinMedica 1 percent retinol, and Skin-Ceuticals 1 percent retinol, among others.

Weekly

I suggest working a weekly mask into your forties skin care routine. There are some nice sleeping masks that are more like a cream. Products like Garnier SkinActive masks are available in a range from pore-cleansing clay masks to hydrating hyaluronic acid and leave your skin hydrated and your pores looking smaller in as little as fifteen minutes. I also like the SkinCeuticals Biocellulose Restorative Masque. It's paraben-free and great for sensitive, dry skin.

Bonus Treatments (all of which I've covered throughout the book)

- Neuromodulators

- Ultherapy

- Fractional CO2

- Fillers

- Kybella

THE FABULOUS FIFTIES AND SEXY SIXTIES

"Nature gives you the face you have at twenty; it is up to you to merit the face you have at fifty."

—*Coco Chanel*

The first question I ask my patients in this age-group when they come in for aesthetic treatments is: "What is your primary goal: Do you want to look younger or do you want to look more beautiful?" Many women are seeking to look younger, and they see that as eliminating every line and wrinkle. Looking more beautiful, as you now well understand from reading this book, is the answer I hope you're going for.

Fifty Is the New Fifty!

Newly dubbed the Perennials, women in their fifties have the strongest sense of themselves because they know what they want and what they don't want, which can make this one of the best times in their lives!

At some point, many of us will become grandparents, bringing even more joy into our lives (without the responsibility of full-time child care). Physically, there are changes happening at every structural level, from bone to fat to collagen and elastic tissue in the skin, that affect how we look as we age. We experience a steep drop in hormones after menopause, and the natural signs of aging appear, along with lines that tell of those younger years of tanning and excess. As hormone levels drop, collagen production slows down dramatically, unless you are doing hormone replacement therapy. Moisturizing and hydration become essential to help skin retain its health, elasticity, and radiance.

An outstanding treatment to consider in your fifties is vaginal rejuvenation. There are excellent devices available, such as the FemTouch and Fotona lasers, that are virtually painless and can, in as little as one to three treatments, improve lubrication, reduce incontinence, and enhance sexual pleasure. One of the greatest compliments I got after a treatment was a text from a patient turning seventy: "I just turned 70 and it was better than ever! Thank you, I love you!!" That healthy glow made any treatment we did on her face look even better.

Keep this in mind as you blow out more candles on your birthday cake: Getting older is inevitable; aging is optional. I came up with this tagline after being interviewed for a Barbara Walters 20/20 special titled "The Cutting Edge." I've never met as thoughtful and insightful an interviewer as Barbara, and it was an honor to be selected by her for this special. She cares deeply about her work, and her questions were always spot-on. At the end of the interview she asked me, "Does this mean we never have to get old?" It took me over a year to really figure it out. Finally, it occurred to me that there is a clear and obvious difference between getting older and aging.

Getting older is great because it means we're still here, hopefully wiser and fulfilled in our lives. Aging is another story. There is a difference between your chronological age and your biologic age. You've been here a certain number of years, but that's truly just a number these days. In reality, one person's biologic age can be very different from another's even if they were born the same year. Your lifestyle choices—sun exposure, stress, alcohol, sleep, diet, emotional factors, and more—have a powerful positive or negative impact on how you age, and this really starts to show when you hit your fifties.

When I see patients for an aesthetic consult, the one piece of homework I give them is to find a photo from when they were in their twenties or thirties. This helps me analyze how they have aged and also helps me restore them to their most attractive selves without changing how they look. If I do my job well, the work is invisible, and they look radiant and beautiful without anyone knowing what was done. They might not look twenty or thirty again, but they look beautiful.

For women in their fifties and sixties, beauty is discipline and requires consistency over time. I recommend that they do the following for their skin.

Nightly

Use night cream to combat dryness and crepiness. Facial oils and overnight masks can also help with dryness and crepiness. Drugstore night cream brands I like include Roc and Olay ProX. The prescription products I recommend are SkinMedica Dermal Repair cream, NeoStrata Skin Active Cellular Restoration, Tensage cream with stem cells, SkinCeuticals triple lipid, Skin Better AlphaRet, Regenica, and Tensage Intensive Serum 40.

Bonus Treatments (we've covered these in detail):

- Neuromodulators.

- Fillers. Especially the lifting fillers, often layered with the softer ones.

- Lasers. We can now lower the risk of skin cancer, smooth out wrinkles from sun damage, and even out skin tone with fractional resurfacing lasers and devices.

- Chemical peels. If you have rosacea or sensitive skin, ones with phytic acid are a good place to start.

- Devices and lasers for tightening and contouring of the face and body.

- Kybella.

- Sclerotherapy (for unsightly veins).

ASK DR. DAY

Q: *I've been seeing new night creams for the body. Do I need one, and are they really any different from day creams?*

DD: The skin goes through different processes during the day than it does at night. Oil gland production and water retention are greater during the day, while the night is known to be an important, but still largely poorly understood time for healing for the body, including the skin. Your skin also loses water overnight, and that can leave your skin feeling dry when you wake up in the morning. Skin that is overly dry can be itchy, flaky, and more prone to irritation and infection. The legs have fewer oil glands than other parts of the body so they are naturally drier, and this becomes more of an issue as we age.

Body creams and ointments that offer the greatest hydration usually feel too heavy and greasy to use during the day, especially when you need to get dressed right afterward. The best time to apply is after a lukewarm shower or bath when the skin is still damp. This will help pull water into the skin and lock it in. Ingredients you should look for are shea butter, ceramides, lactic acid, glycerin, antioxidants such as grape seed or green tea extract, and vitamins A, C, and E. Such a rich base provides an environment that is most conducive to the antioxidants' penetration deeper into the skin where they are most needed. Regular lotions and creams have many or all of the same ingredients; however, they are usually formulated to be lighter and may not be as hydrating.

Q: *Is there a supplement that can slow the aging process?*

DD: TA-65MD: Telomeres are a stretch of repetitive DNA sequences located at the end of each chromosome. Every human cell contains ninety-two of these biological ticking clocks. The goal is to keep your telomeres as long as possible for as long as possible. They can be maintained or lengthened by activating an enzyme in our bodies called Telomerase. TA-65 is extracted from the root of a select Chinese adaptogenic herb called Astragalus. The TA-65 compound is blended with USP grade products to ensure consistency, and produced according to GMP standards for dietary supplements. It contains no yeast, dairy, eggs, gluten, corn, soy, wheat, sugar, starch, preservatives, artificial color, flavor, or fragrances. To date, T.A. Sciences has completed seven peer-reviewed clinical trials. The latest published double-blind, placebo-controlled, one-year trial showed a roughly three-year biological age improvement.

MAKEUP THROUGH THE AGES

Emmy award–winning makeup artist Lori Klein says, "Having the right makeup and knowing how to apply it can give a woman newfound confidence. I often see a transformation in my client's personality when they like the way they look. The first thing someone will do when they sit in my chair is tell me about their flaws. Even the most beautiful celebrity client will point out their physical faults, real or imagined. We're so lucky to have the art of makeup to enhance and transform each and every one of us."

The following are some tricks of the trade from Lori for makeup through the decades:

Q: *What are your makeup suggestions for women in their twenties?*

LK: Generally speaking, younger women have tighter skin, but women of all ages start with a primer. I use a nice nude lipstick on a young girl. Gloss is much easier for women in their twenties, so that's a good thing to have in your makeup kit. I'm a big proponent of eyelash curlers, which help make eyes look bigger and make your lashes look especially good when you're younger and your lashes are thicker. It helps, even if you're not wearing makeup. I suggest getting the smaller plastic ones instead of the traditional metal curlers. A brow tamer is also good for women in their twenties because their brows are thicker and that look is really popular now. This is a time of your life when you can get away with going with the trends, such as sparkles or a glossier eye, if you want to. I predict that we are going to move away from the dark, smokey look and go back to natural-looking makeup. A dual-purpose finish powder can work well for young people, as well as a pale shimmer shadow. Go minimal and play up the eyes and lips. Use lighter foundations unless you need to cover up. There are some great concealers out there if you need it for breakouts. Once your skin is clean and prepared with moisturizer, I believe a foundation can protect your skin. If you have oily skin or acne, you should use a water-based foundation. I recommend putting the SPF on first because foundations that contain sunscreen don't have enough in it and it changes the makeup texture. Stila and Urban Decay lines are great for high-shine eye shadow that caters to younger women; when you're younger you can get that glowy look much easier than when you're older.

Q: What are the biggest mistakes women in their twenties make when it comes to makeup?
LK: Wearing too much makeup.

Q: Should a woman in her thirties start using fake lashes or lash extensions?
LK: I did an entire segment on *The View* about eyelashes. There are so many great products out there now, and fake eyelashes are actually great for any age.

Here are the steps:

1. Store-bought eyelashes, which are great, are sometimes too long, so you want to trim them so they fit properly.
2. Next, you want to roll them in your fingers so they fit the natural curve of your eye. Hold one end in each hand and bend it into a curved shape like a Slinky.
3. Apply a thin strip of glue, always nonpermanent, so you can remove them easily. Wait a few seconds to let the glue get tacky before you put the lashes on, continuing to roll them. Waiting for the glue to get tacky is a key step. Tweezers sometimes help to hold lashes when applying.

Q: What is highlighting or strobing?
LK: In your twenties, thirties, and forties you can do what we professionals call highlighting or strobing, which is using a cream or powder to highlight certain areas of the face for contouring. Apply a light color on top of the cheekbones and at the bow of the lip. On the forehead you can place a little shimmering cream or powder. You have to be careful as you get older not to overdo the highlighting.

Q: *What kinds of makeup mistakes do women in their thirties make?*

LK: The biggest mistake I see women in this age-group make is being afraid to try something new. You might want to experiment with some new colors and styles. Try a pencil line outside the eye instead of inside, for instance. Thirties is a time for looking more sophisticated.

Q: *Women in their forties might start seeing gravity take its toll. What are some tips for getting a makeup lift?*

LK: I take a little bit of nude- to pale-colored shadow and after I do makeup I put it on the outside of the eye and under the cheekbone to lift the eye up. I like to extend the liner slightly up and out, under and over the eyes to lift them. This creates an instant lift. Curling the lashes is extremely important now. Try starting with the outside and working your way in. Take a spoolie brush (or dry mascara brush) and brush through your eyelashes before you curl. Always do it before you apply mascara to avoid breakage and clumping. If your lashes are thinning, I like to layer different kinds of mascara. I start with very thin mascara for a more natural look, always using a spoolie brush between the layers to clean up clumps. Then I'd apply volumizing mascara depending on how dramatic you want to go. Applying many layers of mascara might mean you don't need the fake lashes.

Q: *What is your advice for blush and foundation?*

LK: Cream blush is great underneath a powder. As we age we tend to absorb our makeup more and it seems to disappear. My trick as a makeup artist is to stay pale in the blush. Put a little blush underneath the chin and on the cheekbones. The biggest mistake a woman at this age makes is that the blush is too dark or in the wrong place. With foundation, try your best to match your skin tone. When I do my own makeup I use my fingers, but you can also use a brush or a sponge, whatever works for you.

Always make sure that you blend the foundation into the hairline and neckline. Again, a primer really helps make the skin smooth before applying foundation. I like Clarins Instant Smooth or Freeze 24-7 cream. It makes all the little fine lines disappear and smooths out the skin. Put it on after doing your usual skin care regimen.

Q: *What are the special needs and makeup tips for women in their fifties and sixties?*

LK: At this point you have to be careful about using too much makeup. Nobody wants to look like an oil slick, but the products you now use are really important. Do they make your pores look worse or your skin cakey? Don't be afraid of using foundation and powder as long as you get the right formula. So many women come to me and say, "I'm using too much powder," but good powder will smooth out your skin, not dry it out. You have to do a little searching. Finding the right shade of foundation is so important, especially as you get older. It helps to get a makeup lesson or see a professional makeup artist to learn of the best products and ways to apply them for your skin.

Q: *What about lipstick color at this age?*

LK: If you have a beautiful full mouth, you can wear a brighter, stronger lipstick. As we age the lower part of the face gets hard, so accentuate your eyes instead. I don't think there is any reason why a woman in her fifties and sixties can't have dramatic eyes using blacks and silvers; it can look amazing. For thinning and lined lips, use a nude pencil to reshape the lips and make them fuller. Use a lip brush to apply the first layer of lipstick, blot it, and put a little powder on top and apply another layer of lipstick. After you put lip liner on, blend it with your fingers.

Older women need a little color on their lips. Mattes are fine because there are great products out there that don't dry out the lips.

Q: **What makeup should women in this age-group use for their brows?**

LK: Brows will change your appearance at any age. Go to a professional to get help with shaping, then try to re-create what they've done yourself. Go slightly lighter than your own brow color and use a brow powder with an angled brush or a thin brow pencil to fill in sparse areas. Clear gel can set the brows if they are unruly, but you should brush up and trim the long hairs. Stick with brow powders or a brow pencil to fill in sparse areas, and a clear gel on top. I'm not fond of the colored gels because they don't look natural. Stila is an affordable choice.

Q: **What do you recommend for dark circles?**

LK: Put the concealer on first. There are creams and liquids that come in many forms—pots, pens, tubes, even pencils. I'd go with a peachy tone to eliminate the dark circles, or a color slightly lighter than your skin tone. Use it under the foundation and sometimes again over the foundation. Most important is the correct color and texture. I like to test on the inside of my thumb where there are a lot of lines. You can really see if the concealer is going to cover and not cake.

BEAUTIFUL SKIN TRAVELS

Here is some advice for taking your skin care on the road. I've always loved to travel, and if you follow my blog, you'll know I travel a lot for work, mostly by plane, to lecture and serve on advisory boards. As a little girl, my parents would pack up the three kids and take us away as often as my dad could manage around his busy doctor's schedule. The airport itself was an exciting destination alone, and we dressed up for the trip as if we were going to a party. Travel by car or train was just as exciting, and the idea of an adventure always appealed to me—the feeling has never worn off. It may have something to do with the fact that I still live in the same city, and even in the same building where I was born and raised, so I have the comfort and security of knowing where home is and that makes a new place, hotel, and scene intriguing. Or maybe it's just me.

Adjusting to Time Zones. The thing about travel that can be the most challenging is dealing with the havoc it wreaks on the skin. Totally not acceptable. Sounds superficial, I know, but I know it's more than just skin-deep. When I see tired, travel-worn skin, I know there's way more going on below the surface and adjustments that need to be made to stay healthy in mind, body, and skin in order to make the entire trip more productive and fun.

When traveling to different time zones, try to transition to that time zone during the flight by planning nap and awake times and adjusting the light to help you acclimate even before you arrive. Try to pick flights that optimize the process. It takes a little planning but makes all the difference in minimizing jet lag and getting the most out of the trip. This way you hit the ground running and can be the most productive when you arrive.

Staying Hydrated. Hydration is key. This means more water, less salt, and less alcohol. I said it was important; I didn't say it was fun. I also said less, not none. The longer the trip, the more important this is. I've seen people whose feet and ankles swell to three or more times their size, and that can take days to resolve. Wearing compression socks can help, along with leg elevation when possible, walking around during the flight, or stopping to walk if you're in a car, and also doing flex and point foot exercises when sitting. And of course, I repeat, more water, less alcohol, less salt.

Packing for Your Skin. Preparing your skin for travel starts even before you leave the house. If you're a last-minute packer, I recommend making a skin care travel kit that's always ready to go. Most of us notice that our skin gets dry when we travel, and if you're prone to eczema or psoriasis, this can trigger a flare. It's especially important to have a great moisturizer to keep your skin healthy and hydrated. Drinking water won't make the outer layers less dry, so you need to moisturize and hydrate the skin directly. If you have oily skin and break out, the stress of traveling can trigger an episode, leaving you both oily and dehydrated at the same time. It's not always easy to pack all your acne medications when you travel, but it is important to maintain your routine to minimize any breakouts when you least want one.

ON-THE-GO ESSENTIALS

The one thing you need to coordinate and organize ahead of time is a travel skin care kit so you can avoid any skin catastrophes that might ruin your trip.

Carry-On (Travel Size)

- Hand cream: It can also be used on the body as needed.

- Premoistened cleansing cloths: Test the brand ahead of time and look for one with cloths that are softer rather than abrasive on the skin.

- Sunscreen: A good tinted sunscreen can double as a foundation for travel purposes.

- Lip balm: Airplane air is drying to the skin and even more drying to the lips. A good lip balm will help keep your lips hydrated and soft.

- Tissues: Always good to keep handy.

- Nail file: Dry air on the plane and trauma from lifting bags and opening wrappers of food and drink can lead to broken nails. The sharp surfaces are uncomfortable and encourage nail biting to smooth the edges. Carrying a nail file will help smooth the nail out and avoid snags on clothing from the rough edges.

- Hair tie/scrunchy: They may be out of vogue for public use, but they are perfect to keep your hair off your face on a long flight or car ride without pulling or stressing your hair.

- Antiperspirant: This can also be used in the groin and between the thighs to prevent chafing or sweating if you're traveling to hot, humid climates.

- Airplane socks: A travel luxury, yet totally necessary. You can buy them at any drugstore and enjoy warm, soft, comfortable feet on the plane or in the car.

- Eye covers and earplugs: Nothing says beautiful skin better than a good night's sleep, or a nap on the plane in this case (the baby screaming behind me was barely audible once my earplugs were in). Tip: Noise-canceling headphones are good but may not be as comfortable for sleeping.

- Toothbrush and toothpaste: Use bottled water to rinse. Most airplane bathroom water is not drinkable.

- Avène water spray: Mist your face to add hydration every hour or so when you're awake on the plane, on the train, or in the car.

Final Thoughts

What I've observed through my twenty years of practice is that beauty is as much a feeling, an expression, and about living life to its fullest as it is physically related to your skin. My greatest fulfillment comes from learning about and helping my patients see the best in themselves, and to bring that to the surface, so what they see in the mirror is a reflection of their true beauty. This transcends youth and makes it possible to look even more beautiful with every decade, for as long as we are fortunate enough to be on this earth.

I've learned so much from seeing patients, from studying medicine, and from traveling the world lecturing and sharing information with colleagues. I've also learned from my own life experiences, and it has been my pleasure and privilege to share what I've learned with you. I hope that you, like me, can learn to accept yourself and be yourself, laugh at your quirks, and celebrate your strengths.

My last piece of advice to you is to try to compartmentalize and keep what's important at the top, never compare yourself to anyone else, and be sure to help and elevate those around you as much as you can. This isn't always easy, but the challenges make us better. Continuously push yourself out of your comfort zone to grow, learn, and become better at what you do and to be as fulfilled in life as possible. The work you do on the inside and how you feel about yourself as a result will radiate beautifully from your face.

I have had many of the treatments I've discussed here in this book, and I've outlined them for you with confidence, but I've also done my best to aim for balance in my own skin care and aesthetic treatments. I celebrate each day, I don't take a minute of it for granted, and I encourage you to do the same.

I have loved sharing my thoughts and ideas with you. I hope you are able to benefit and make every day your #bestDAYever.

"Could a greater miracle take place than for us to look through each other's eyes for an instant?"

—Henry David Thoreau

Acknowledgments

Thank you to...

My patients for your faith in me and for trusting me with your health, beauty, and wellness and for sharing your lives with me. It is my greatest privilege and honor to be your doctor and my mission is to always put you first.

My daughter, Sabrina Adriane, my best friend and my best editor. Thank you for keeping me focused and helping me write the best book possible. I'm so proud of you; you are so well prepared for medical school and a brilliant career in medicine. I hope this book serves you well as you continue on your journey. To Kambiz Ghalili, my husband and soul mate of nearly thirty years, and my brilliant son, Andrew, thank you for being the best family ever. And thank you to my mom, Shekoofeh Day, for always being my biggest cheerleader and fan.

Kent Remington, thank you for adopting me into your fold and always sharing your brilliant insights, creative ideas, and pushing me beyond my comfort zone to become better and better at my craft.

Arthur Swift, so many of my creative thoughts and writings have come to me after hearing you speak and watching you teach. I have learned so much from you my King (of aesthetics). Arturo, nothing makes me prouder than when you call me Queen!

I am blessed to have a family of Derm Diva Sisters with whom I can share ideas, thoughts, and patient cases, and, of course, fashion and shopping plans. I thank each and every one of you for being part of such a supportive group. We will grow old together, looking our very best and better every year.

Thank you to the brilliant Jane Greer for being a shining light and for being my angel sister of the heart.

My thanks to my producer, Jessica Bari, to listeners of SiriusXM Doctor Radio, and to followers on social media. Many of the stories and ideas for this book were developed and grew from conversations on radio.

My thanks to dear friends and brilliant thinkers, philanthropists, writers, and confidants who inspire me and always make me want to do more: Caroline Kimmel, Francine LeFrak, Donna Tartt, Paula Zahn, Rachel Weintraub Riegel, Rob Wallace, Whoopi Goldberg, and Nicolle Wallace.

Index

About the Author

Doris Day, MD, is a board certified dermatologist specializing in aesthetic and laser in New York City. Dr. Day is a clinical associate professor of dermatology at the New York University Langone Medical Center. She has won awards for her work in laser research, teaching, and for promoting her specialty of dermatology.

Dr. Day regularly lectures at aesthetic conferences worldwide. She is a member of several national and international organizations including the American Society for Dermatologic Surgery, the American Academy of Dermatology, the Women's Dermatologic Society, the Dermatologic Society of Greater New York, and New York Facial Plastic Surgery Society. She has been elected by her peers to serve on the board of directors for the ASDS and also serves as chair of the media committee. She is also an inductee into the American Honors Society of Dental and Facial Aesthetics and has served on the medical advisory boards and training panels for Allergan, Galderma, and Merz, among others.

Dr. Day has published many peer reviewed articles and chapters on aesthetics and is the author of three books, *Beyond Beautiful*, *Forget the Facelift*, and *100 Questions & Answers About Acne*. She regularly appears on national television shows and is the famed host of an award-winning show on the Doctor Radio channel on SiriusXM 110.

Dr. Day earned an English degree from Columbia University, her masters in journalism and science writing at New York University, and her MD at Downstate Medical School in New York. She completed her residency in Dermatology at Cornell University College of Medicine with the title of chief resident. She and her husband of nearly thirty years have two grown children, Andrew and Sabrina.

Dr. Day invites you to visit her website, www.myclearskin.com, where you can read her blog, or follow her on Instagram, Facebook, Twitter, and Snapchat @DrDorisDay. You can also listen to her or call her on Doctor Radio. She'll be happy to answer all of your questions, cheer you on, and help you to become the best and most beautiful version of yourself—inside and out!